48 DOG-FRIENDLY TRAILS

in California's Foothills and the Sierra Nevada

DEBBI PRESTON

authorHOUSE®

AuthorHouse™
1663 Liberty Drive, Suite 200
Bloomington, IN 47403
www.authorhouse.com
Phone: 1-800-839-8640

First published by AuthorHouse 7/2/2008

ISBN: 978-1-4343-7766-1 (sc)

Library of Congress Control Number: 2008905162

Printed in the United States of America
Bloomington, Indiana

This book is printed on acid-free paper.

Cover photo: Jeff Preston, 2007   View from top of Mt. Tallac

Edited by Pamela Preston

ACKNOWLEDGEMENTS

I sincerely thank my husband, Jeff, for accompanying me on so many of these hikes, and for encouraging me to write this book Also, a huge thanks to my dog, Toots, for always being with me, eager to go hiking.

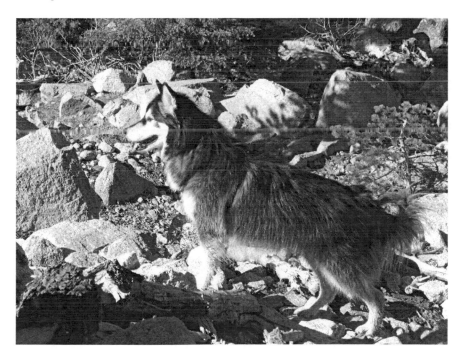

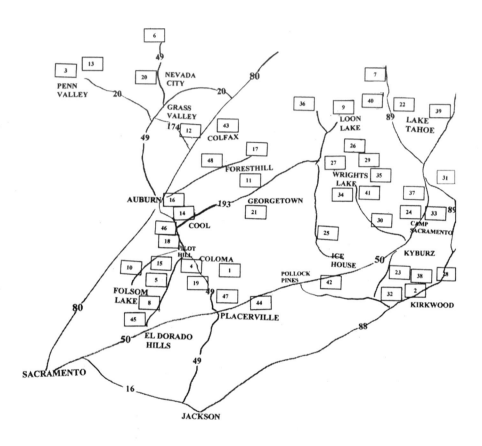

TABLE OF CONTENTS

MAY

JUNE

JULY

AUGUST

SEPTEMBER

OCTOBER

NOVEMBER

DECEMBER

Trail Essentials and Wisdom

Hiking requires common sense and the acceptance of its many risks. While the hikes in this book are associated with certain months, in some years, the weather may be such that there are late seasonal storms, so the June hikes are not reachable until late July. Also, there could be early storms, preventing certain hikes scheduled for October and November. In 2006, with the heavy winter rains and snow, Maud Lake was not reachable on my first attempt in late June, as the Jones Fork Silver Creek crossing was too dangerous. In 2007, a light rain year, I made this hike easily in mid-June. Be willing to turn back if conditions exist to make going forward dangerous.

Furthermore, while I have made great effort to detail trail routes, signs can change over the years, trails renamed, markers added, and sometimes posts once there can now be missing. It is essential that you carry a good map and perhaps a pedometer to mark your mileage. Then, if a sign has changed or is missing, you can still refer to the trail description of distances, and to your trail map, to verify your path choice.

Do not attempt a trail too difficult for your abilities, unless you are willing to turn around once out of your comfort zone. Allow plenty of time for your hike, and turn back if you cannot complete the journey before dark. Most importantly, be safe and enjoy.

Items essential in your pack:

1. First aid kit and pocketknife
2. Map
3. Hat
4. Ample water for you and for your dog
5. Ample food, enough for an extra day if needed
6. Whistle and flashlight (with extra batteries)
7. Insect repellant
8. Sun screen
9. Layered clothing
10. Waterproof matches and flint (fires are not allowed in Desolation Wilderness except in the case of an emergency)

Also good to bring along:

1. Sunglasses
2. Camera
3. Trail book/Wildflower book (in season)
4. Watch
5. Walking poles
6. Spare socks
7. Small fold-up shovel
8. Toilet paper
9. Plastic bag for dog leavings; leash
10. Pedometer

Trail Wisdom and Etiquette:

1. Let someone know where you are going and when you will return.
2. Yield to uphill hikers and to all equestrians and pack animals.
3. Pick up or bury any dog leavings.
4. Do not allow your dog to bother the wildlife or other hikers.
5. When arriving at a lake, always note the trail in, and look for markers to remind you of your path later when you are ready to leave.
6. Do not continue on an unclear trail until you can see your next marker or other sure sign of the trail.
7. Do not attempt a trail above your hiking abilities.
8. Do not rush; always make sure of your footing to avoid injury.
9. Turn back if thunderstorms threaten.
10. Allow plenty of time for your hike to avoid darkness (dusk brings out more wild animals, so be sure to be back to your car well before then).

Trail Planning

Hiking is an extremely popular and healthy exercise option, requiring little equipment or expense, while rewarding our bodies with overall fitness. Hiking is linked with lowering blood pressure, reducing stress, and lowering bad cholesterol levels. With hiking, you visit many new places to see and to learn about, and mostly to enjoy. Obviously there are risks with natural elements, wild animals, poison oak, ticks, mosquitoes, and injuries, but if you take the time to study where you will be hiking, inform others of your plans, and only go forward when you are sure of the trail and your capabilities, then you should minimize these risks.

All of the following hikes are day hikes, local enough to Sacramento for you to accomplish in a day. These are also all dog-friendly adventures. Many are especially good for children, with interpretive trails for learning and visits to historical sites. Some hikes are good for those with physical disabilities, but still desiring an outdoor experience. Each month there will be an option for the physically challenged, or for those just starting an exercise program.

The month selected for a hike is to optimize the experience. For instance, you visit waterfalls when they will be at their peak. You journey in the spring to foothill locations to enjoy the wildflowers, and then leave for higher elevations to avoid the valley's summer heat.

Furthermore, you will visit places when they will not be as crowded whenever possible.

I rate trails in difficulty from '1' (easiest) to '5' (hardest). I base the rating on a combination of mileage, terrain, feet climbed, and difficulty in reading the trail. A trail rating of '1' is equal to walking around a high school track, with just a little elevation change. A '2' rating is usually a longer hike, and more elevation change, but still not strenuous. A '3' rating indicates some difficulty and a need for a moderate fitness level. The hikes are longer, with some tough climbs, and the trails are not always well marked. A '4' rating will require a great deal of climbing and trail reading ability. These are only suited to the more physically fit. A '5' rating will be a strenuous hike, with extreme climbs, and trail reading difficulty.

The elevation gain is generally from the lowest point on the trail to the highest or from the trailhead parking to the destination. The information is for your reference before starting the hike, to help you determine if the hike is suitable for you. In some cases, the gain can be misleading if there are many "ups and downs" on the trail. For instance, the Maud Lake hike gains only 640 feet from the parking area to the lake; however, the trail first goes uphill, then down to a creek, and then back up again. Therefore, the overall climb in total vertical feet is greater than the elevation gain.

For mountain hikes, a good topographical map of the area will help you to see ahead of time how difficult it may be. A topographical map shows the contours of the terrain. Every 40-foot elevation change has a contour line, with a darker line every 200 feet. Therefore, the denser the lines are, the steeper the grade. If you climb 500 feet over a mile distance, it is easy when compared to climbing 500 feet in 0.25 mile. Therefore, if the elevation gain is covering a greater distance on a hike, it may still be doable for you. A quick glance at a topographical map will let you see if there are any difficult sections (closer contour lines) in your proposed trip.

Day-use permits are required for all hikes entering into Desolation Wilderness. The permits are free, and in most instances available at the trailheads from July until October of each year. After the end of the general hiking season in October, you need to pick up a permit at one of the ranger stations. On Highway 50 in Fresh Pond, you take the Mill Run exit to reach the Pacific Ranger District and obtain a permit. They do not need to be open for you to get the permit, since they have a supply in a box outside of their offices.

JANUARY

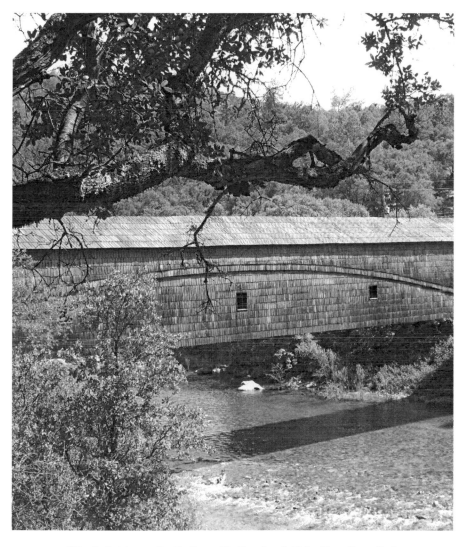

Wood's Bridge on Pt. Defiance Trail at South Yuba River State Park

JANUARY

While winter looms in the mountains, there are still places in the foothills to explore in more pleasant weather. For those who enjoy the snow and have 4-wheel drive vehicles, there are snowshoeing opportunities as well. January is the perfect time to start an exercise program and these first hikes start you off easily.

This month you visit the Marshall Gold Discovery State Historic Park in Coloma during a quiet tourist time. This is a flat walk (unless you choose to walk up to the monument), so it is good for people with physical disabilities. It is also good for children to learn about the early gold mining times, with many replicas and signs describing the items from the mid 1800's. You visit the sight where the longest existing covered bridge in the United States is on the Pt. Defiance hike in the South Yuba River State Park as well. You try out snowshoeing in Kirkwood and then enjoy the least busy time at Cronan Ranch with a hike down to the South Fork American River.

Hike 1 - Marshall Gold Discovery State Historic Park
Coloma, CA

Difficulty: 1 (or 2 if you hike up Monument Road)
Distance: 3.0 miles (including hike up to Monument)
Elevation: Flat, except for 200-foot ascent up Monument Road

Directions: From Highway 50 in Shingle Springs, take the Ponderosa Road exit and go north across the freeway. After crossing the freeway, turn right onto North Shingle Road at the light immediately after the signal for the westbound off-ramp (signed Lotus, Coloma, Georgetown, Rescue, No. Shingle Rd.). North Shingle Road merges with and becomes Green Valley Road after 4.0 miles. In 0.4 miles, Green Valley Road veers to the right. Stay straight here and you will now be on Lotus Road. In 6.8 miles, Lotus Road will dead end at Highway 49.

Turn right towards Coloma at the three-way stop where Lotus Road ends at Highway 49. Just outside the state park boundaries, within 0.1 mile, there is a parking area on the river's side of the highway at the yellow blinking light for the stop ahead. This is a free parking area, unlike the parking within the park itself. If you do not want to walk from the outskirts of the park, continue on Highway 49 and park in one of the fee parking areas.

Description: This is a fun, informational hike, especially for families. You enjoy a pleasant walk and can learn a great deal about California's early settlers.

After parking, start walking along the river's side of Highway 49. In a short distance, you will find a spur trail (a spur is a narrow footpath off a main trail without any markings) taking you off the road and into the park. You can walk through the park and find a path along the river. This path has many stopping points with historical markers giving you information about this site where James Marshall first discovered gold in California. There is also a replica of the sawmill Marshall and his workers used, as well as other historic buildings, cabin replicas, representative shops, and displays. You can cross the iron bridge to the other side of the river, but dogs are not allowed on the trail on that side.

After the bridge, continue to the end of the street where you can see the old Coloma Schoolhouse. Here you need to make the decision to walk up to the Marshall Monument or to drive up there after completing a tour of the park on the other side. The walk up to the monument will be a 200-foot ascent.

If you decide to walk, then cross the road and walk up Highway 49 for 0.1 mile to where the highway will curve away to the left. If you continue straight, however, you will be on Cold Springs Road. Walk up Cold Springs Road 0.1 mile to Monument Road, then turn right onto Monument Road and go 0.4 mile to reach the parking area at the base of the monument. You can go up the steps to the monument and look down across to the sites below, reminiscent of an old mining town. From the monument, find the road to Marshall's cabin. This road winds you down the hill to the old cabin, the Catholic Cemetery, and St. John's Church. You will end up in the park again heading towards the Visitor Center. Continue your walk along this side of the park back to your car.

There is a lot to see here and to read at each exhibit. Numerous picnic areas are available as well. There are two hiking trails, the Monument Trail and Monroe Ridge Trail, but dogs are not allowed on either one. Plan to spend a lot of time here even though the mileage is short. Remember to drive up to the monument if you did not hike there.

For information about events throughout the year in the park, visit www.marshallgold.org or call 530-295-2162. For a walking map, go to www.parks.ca.gov.

After the hike: After your stay at the park, you can consider a 0.9 mile drive up Cold Springs Road to **Gold Hill Winery** for free wine tasting. They are open Thursday-Sunday, from 10:00 to 5:00.

Hike 2 - Kirkwood, CA
Cross Country & Snowshoe Center

Difficulty: 1-2 with easy to moderate options

Distance: Varies, depending on trails selected

Elevation: Base elevation is 7800' with 80 kilometers (about 48 miles) of groomed trails, ranging from Easiest, Intermediate, to Advanced so elevation gains vary

Warnings: There are fees for using the groomed trails and for renting equipment. Waterproof your boots ahead of time, and bring a change of shoes and socks in case your feet get wet.

Description: This is a fun outing for the whole family, including your dog (on the dog-friendly designated trails). Drive 60 miles east of Jackson on Highway 88 to reach Kirkwood. The ski resort is on your right, but continue past it a very short distance to find the Cross Country & Snowshoe Center on your left. Here you can purchase your pass and get a map of the various trails. If it is your first time to snowshoe, consider doing the half-day adventure starting at 1:00pm. Get there ahead of time and enjoy a lunch on their deck, while planning your route for the day.

The trails are well marked, with all distances noted in kilometers (compute to approximate miles by multiplying by 0.6). Please note that the only rules for your dog are to stay on designated trails and to pick up any waste in order to keep the trails pristine (leashes **not** required). There is one dog-friendly trail marked easy, two are intermediate, and one has an advanced rating, so there is plenty of opportunity awaiting you. Bring your camera for capturing plenty of gorgeous views and documenting the fun time enjoyed by your family.

Notes: Watch for **Winter Trails Day** for an opportunity to try out a number of snowshoes from various vendors, get guided equipment and shoeing instruction, and a fun day – all at no cost. Visit **kirkwood.com** for details and dates.

Trail Pass Rates				**Snowshoe Rentals**		
	All Day	½ Day (1 pm)			All Day	½ Day
Adult	$22.00	18.00		Adult	$22.00	18.00
13-18	17.00	15.00		Child	10.00	8.00
65+	17.00	15.00				
70+	12.00	12.00				
11-12	8.00	8.00				
Dog	4.00					
Ten and under free						

Above prices are for 2007/08. Phone (209)258-7248 for updates.

Hike 3 - Pt. Defiance Trail to Englebright Lake
South Yuba River State Park
Bridgeport, CA

Difficulty: 2
Distance: 2.8-mile loop
Elevation: 380-foot climb

Warnings: *Respect the park's rules about dogs not allowed on the beach areas along the river in the immediate park area. Also, note limited access May-September for dogs.*

Directions: In Grass Valley, from Highway 49, take the exit for Highway 20 to Marysville and Penn Valley. Go 7.8 miles on Highway 20 into Penn Valley and turn right onto Pleasant Valley Road. Travel 7.8 miles to the South Yuba River State Park. Parking is on your left near the visitor center.

Description: This is a fun hike, especially for your dog, with lots of opportunities to run down to the river for a splash. For the naturalist, you walk through a variety of habitats, starting with foothill chaparral and oaks, then canyon buckeyes and madrones, and then the riparian river habitat of willows and cottonwoods. For the historian, the park features one of only ten covered bridges remaining in California.

Starting from the parking lot, you walk across the covered bridge. This bridge, called Wood's Bridge, is the longest existing covered bridge in the United States. Built in 1862, it spans 251 feet across the South Fork Yuba River.

After crossing the bridge, turn right and walk along the service road, cross another service road, and immediately find the trailhead pointing 1.7 miles to Pt. Defiance.

This first part of the trail consists of switchbacks taking you up a 380-foot hill lush with native brush and oaks. At the top, there is a picnic table for a short break. Continuing on the trail, you walk through a meadow, cross a bridge, and then arrive at a service gate. (A service gate crosses wide paths to limit access to service and emergency vehicles only. A number of trailheads start at such a gate that you simply walk around to gain entrance. Never park in front of any gate in and block its access to authorized vehicles).

Walk around the gate and continue down the service road, getting views of Englebright Lake and the Yuba River Canyon on your right. This is a steep descent and can be slippery if wet, so take care on the way down. You bottom out at the confluence of the river and the lake, and a small picnic area shaded by willows. Here you can sit and watch any boaters as you take a break. There are tables and toilet facilities here.

Continuing the loop, the trail narrows as it parallels the river. You can reach the river to try some gold panning at a number of spur trails. The last part of the trail offers you splendid views of the covered bridge before you return across it. Take time to look into the visitor center (open Thursday – Sunday from 11:00 am to 5:00 pm) and enjoy the rest of the park and its history before returning home.

Notes: Plan to return here in early spring when you do Hike 13 – Buttermilk Bend. On the Pt. Defiance loop, spring will bring an array of blue-purple wildflowers, such as blue dick, bush lupine, bowel-tube iris, and larkspur. Also, look for a small grouping of California Indian pink along the service road descent. In this same area, you will also find both the California Pipe Vine and Manroot (wild cucumber vine).

Hike 4 - Cronan Ranch
Pilot Hill, CA

Difficulty: 3 (or 2 depending on option taken)

Distance: 4.8-mile loop (or optional 4.4)

Elevation: 500 feet from lowest to highest point; one
ascent of 400 feet on longer loop

Directions: On Highway 49, coming from Coloma, 5 miles from the bridge crossing the South Fork American River, turn left onto Pedro Hill Road. Coming from Auburn, make a right turn 1.0 mile south of Pilot Hill onto Pedro Hill Road.

A large parking area is a short distance from here towards the left. Try to leave the larger parking spaces for horse trailers and park near the map at the start of the trailhead or along the exit road. (For more detailed directions, see Hike 1.)

Description: The Cronan Ranch offers trails throughout its 1,418 acres, open to hikers, mountain bikers, and equestrians. Once private ranch property, it is now public and run by the Bureau of Land Management (BLM). The trails are well marked with directional signs, but the markers do not give the trail names that you find on the map at the trailhead, making for a little confusion.

Starting beyond the parking area, walk up the hill on Ranch Road for .025 mile and then turn left onto the Down and Up Trail. After another 0.5 mile, the trail comes to an intersection – go right here. Continue a short 0.15 mile to another intersection. Again, go right, putting you onto Hidden Valley Trail.

Follow on Hidden Valley 0.8 mile where it ends at a junction. Turn left here, and now your trail starts to parallel and offer you glimpses of the South Fork American River. Following this "main" trail, you will soon come to two different spur trails taking you down to the river (the second of the spurs is marked 'Trail'). Take either (or both) of these down to the river. While not a great beach, it provides a good resting spot and water hole for your dog (there are portable toilets at both locations).

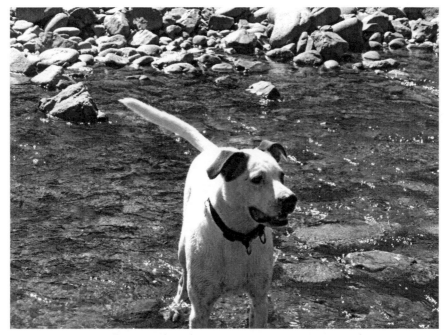

Apollo at South Fork American River in Cronan Ranch

Water levels fluctuate on the river suddenly with frequent water releases for kayakers. My friends visited here and for their lunch break at the river did some rock hopping out to a little island. Within a half hour, the water had risen, making a rock hop back to shore impossible. It was a dangerous walk through the water and they had to rescue their dog when the river swept it away. So be aware of the water levels at all times.

For the trip back, return to the "main" trail and turn right to start the loop back. Along the way, you will pass through a break in fencing marked with a '5'. This is soon followed by a trail off to your left. This is the East Ridge Trail and a shortcut back. (East Ridge offers a couple of picnic tables and vistas along the way before rejoining Hidden Valley Trail and the route back.) For the longer, and tougher, option, continue ahead past this point, now on the aptly named Down & Up Trail.

You will make some 200-foot "ups and downs" along the oak-shaded trail before coming to a small stream lined with blackberries. This is a nice resting spot before continuing again uphill. This next stretch is tough, with a 400-foot elevation gain. Avoid any turns you see along the way, staying straight to the top of the hill. At the top, there is a right turn that would take you to Hastings Creek. Stay straight to rejoin the original trail and the return to the parking area.

Share with: Bikers and horses

After the hike: Go south on Highway 49 for 1.5 miles to find **Venezio Winery** on your left. They offer free wine tasting Wednesday – Sunday, from 11:00 to 5:00.

FEBRUARY

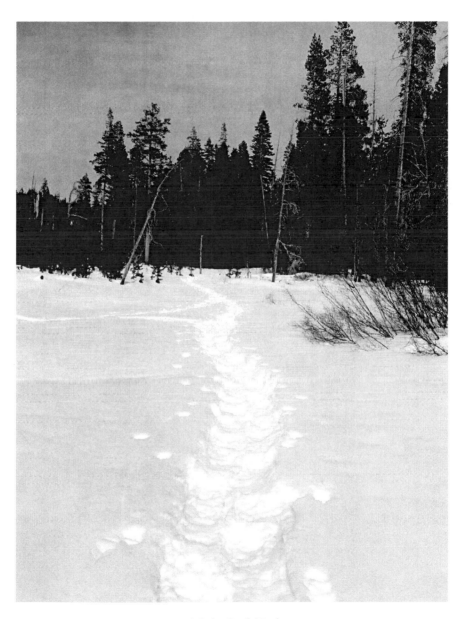

Meeks Creek Trail

FEBRUARY

If you enjoyed snowshoeing in Kirkwood, then you will like this month's choice of Meeks Creek. The whole family should enjoy this nice, flat, route. If the snow has not been heavy this year, you could also try this trail in hiking boots, if you do not have snowshoes. For those with physical disabilities, try the Sweetwater Creek Trail. If you do not have a lot of time to spend a whole day hiking, the Old Salmon Falls Loop is an excellent choice. Farther away, on the Purdon Crossing hike, you visit the only remaining steel bridge in California of the half-truss design.

Hike 5 - Sweetwater Creek Trail
El Dorado Hills, CA
Folsom Lake State Recreation Area

Difficulty: 1

Distance: 2.5 miles to boat launch

Elevation: Very flat, with 10-foot undulations; at most a 30-foot change in elevation (except the last 0.25 mile is more challenging)

Directions: In El Dorado Hills, where El Dorado Hills Boulevard crosses Green Valley Road, it becomes Salmon Falls Road. Drive 3.8 miles on Salmon Falls to find the small parking area on your left (with room for about eight cars). The trailhead starts when you walk past the white service gate.

Description: This is as flat as trails get in the foothills – a good beginner trail for both hikers and mountain bikers. Start through the service gate and shortly there will be a couple of Y's in the trail. Stay to the right at each one and you will be on the signed Sweetwater Trail. At first, the trail follows along Sweetwater Creek and then veers away to follow along the South Fork American River. Continue as far as you like and take one of the many spurs down to the river. The complete trail goes 2.5 miles and ends at the boat launch before Salmon Falls Bridge.

On your return trip, walk down to Sweetwater Creek and pick up a lesser trail that follows along the creek back to the trailhead. Stay to the right with any trail options, staying along the creek as long as possible before returning to your car. On the trail along the creek, you will cross two ditches. In a light rain year, one will most likely be dry and the other an easy rock hop. With a heavy rain, these may be difficult to cross, so you may need to stay on the main Sweetwater Trail on your return.

When water levels are low, you can explore the beaches below the trail and find the remains of buildings, once part of the town of Salmon Falls, an old Mormon gold mining town.

Share with: Bikers

Hike 6 - South Yuba Trail
Purdon Crossing
South Yuba River State Park

Difficulty: 2

Distance: About 4.0 miles to Edwards Crossing, including spur trails down to the river (Trail sign says 4.5 miles to Edwards Crossing, but my pedometer registered less)

Elevation: Undulating trail with 300-feet overall gain, mostly 10-20 foot "ups and downs", with a couple 40-foot climbs mixed in

Directions: In Nevada City, at the split between Highways 49 and 20, turn left to remain on Highway 49 in the direction of Downieville. Go just 0.4 mile and turn right onto N. Bloomfield Road. Go 0.5 mile on N. Bloomfield, and turn left onto Lake Vera Road in the direction of Purdon Crossing. Travel on Lake Vera-Purdon Road for 5.6 miles; the last 1.6 miles section is unpaved and bumpy. At the bottom of the road, you enter South Yuba River State Park with Purdon Bridge on your left. Continue straight into the park (do not cross the bridge) and find the parking area for the trailhead to South Yuba Trail.

Description: Consider bringing your gold pan for this scenic walk along the South Fork Yuba River. On the South Yuba Trail, you will be walking upstream with the river always on your left. You will soon forget the bumpy ride, once you start hiking on this beautiful shaded trail, in a forest of oaks, madrones, buckeyes, pines, and cedars.

The undulating trail takes you along the canyon of the South Fork Yuba River, with the river usually in sight and always within hearing. You will cross numerous streams along the way, and a number of spur trails are available to take you down to the river for a close-up of huge boulders and the clear, green, rushing waters of the Yuba River.

At any trail choice, always choose the uphill option to continue towards Edwards Crossing. The only exception is the uphill choice clearly marked for Round Mountain. After the first 2.5 miles, you exit the shade and the trail becomes rocky, but the views down to the river are striking. Continue about another 1.5 miles to the bridge at Edwards Crossing. Here you will no doubt see gold panners in action. There are toilet facilities here as well as beach areas for lunching before your return trip.

Before leaving the park, be sure to walk across Purdon Bridge. The steel bridge once was used by miners en route from Nevada City to Downieville. Built in 1895, it is the only remaining steel bridge in California built with a half-through truss design.

This is a pretty spring hike also, but the poison oak lining the trail will leaf out then, and the ticks will be thriving as well. You will have a great display of wildflowers later in the season, and rafters to watch, so Purdon Crossing may be well worth a return visit.

Share with: Bikers and horses

Hike 7 - Meeks Creek Trail
Meeks Bay, CA

Difficulty: 1-3, depending on snow conditions

Distance: 2-4 miles, depending on existing tracks

Elevation: Flat trail, 200' gain

Directions: At the "Y" in South Lake Tahoe, leave Highway 50 as it turns to the right (becoming Lake Tahoe Blvd.), and stay straight on Highway 89 towards Tahoe City. Go 16.2 miles on Highway 89 to Meeks Bay and find the parking area on your left.

There is a Forest Service board at the trailhead with information and trail permits for Desolation Wilderness (not necessary for this hike). From the parking area, locate the green forest gate that leads you onto Forest Road 14N32 for the start of the trail.

Description: Your experience will vary depending on the amount of snow. If it is a light snow year, then this will be an easy hike. Make sure to waterproof your hiking boots before starting out and carry a spare pair of socks and shoes in your vehicle to change into at hike's end. You share this trail with cross-country skiers. It is trail etiquette to avoid walking in the ski tracks.

If heavy powder conditions exist, then you will need snowshoes for this adventure and the hike will be more strenuous. You will have to rely mostly on existing tracks for the hike, and you may not find any tracks taking you to Meeks Creek.

Ideally, you will be able to make it to the creek. The trail starts along the service road, continuing straight at first, and then veering left when you approach a hill at the west end of the meadow. Continue on the path following alongside this hill. You are now heading south in the direction of the creek. At 1.4 miles, there will be a marked trail to the right leading into Desolation Wilderness. Stay straight here to continue along the road.

If you manage to stay on the trail, then you will pass by remains of an old camp. The stone foundation remains, along with discarded items like doors and bed frames, and you can imagine what living there would have been like. Climb up the remaining stairs and share the views of the past inhabitants.

The creek lies straight ahead, but depending on the snow and existing tracks, your path may curve back east, making a possible loop back to the trailhead. If you find yourself heading back towards the trailhead, then look for existing tracks going to the right. Follow these back south, if possible, and reach the creek for an enjoyable lunch spot.

The hike is through a meadow, surrounded by hills on three sides, and Highway 89 on the fourth end. The creek is on the south end of the meadow. Whether or not you find your way to the creek, this is an enjoyable outing and a great way to experience snowshoeing. Other popular spots exist along Highway 89 before reaching Meeks Bay, so this is a less crowded location. You may only encounter a few other people at this spot, so you are better able to enjoy the sights and nature's sounds. Plan to revisit in the summer when the trail will be easier to follow without a snowy covering.

Hike 8 - Old Salmon Falls Loop
El Dorado Hills, CA

Difficulty: 1
Distance: 2.2-mile loop
Elevation: 225 feet gain

Warning: *Wear long pants for poison oak along trail*

Directions: From Highway 50 in El Dorado Hills, take the El Dorado Hills Boulevard exit north and go 4.2 miles to Green Valley Road. Continue straight across Green Valley Road and the street becomes Salmon Falls Road. Drive 2.9 miles on Salmon Falls to the large parking area on your left, signed Falcon Crest. Park here and walk down the paved park road signed Folsom State Recreation Area – Old Salmon Falls (parking at the actual trailhead has a fee and since you are doing a loop you would still have to walk down the road to return to your car if you park there).

At the end of the park road (now gravel), you will find the fee parking area on your left. Beyond the parking area, you will find the start of the Brown's Ravine Trail with a marker giving you the distances to the various spots along this route. The entire length of the trail takes you 17.5 miles to Folsom Dam. Starting at the 17.5 mile marker, you are going to do just a portion of this trail.

Description: The first part is a narrow, star thistle-lined trail, bordering private property (I would not look forward to this in summer shorts). Soon the trail climbs uphill away from the residences, giving you a view of the South Fork American River on your right as you make the 100-foot ascent. At the crest of the hill, you can look down to the site of the former mining town of Salmon Falls. Within a mile, you enter a grove of pines planted in 1972, and the thistle disappears, replaced with fresh pine needles and shade. Now it is a pleasant journey, with the trail coming closer to the water.

Just beyond the 16.0-mile marker, you will see a trail junction. You will turn left here to head back to the trailhead. First, though, make a side trip down to the water to enjoy the beach for a while and watch the occasional boat passing by. After your break, return to the junction and follow in the direction to Monte Vista (do not go in the direction of Brown's Ravine).

Leaving Brown's Ravine Trail (and the mile markers), you will walk on a wider trail while enjoying the oak trees. Follow the signs to Potable Water, making a left and a brief ascent of 75 feet. At the top of the small hill, you will reach a picnic area with tables, drinking water, and a trash can (best to pack out your own trash). This spot has a nice view of the surrounding hills and pricey homes.

As you leave the picnic area, look ahead for a green trail marker down the hill towards the left of a dirt road. From the marker, you will again see the trail (if you do not find the marker, you will continue down the dirt road towards Monte Vista South). Stay on the Monte Vista North trail for a quick return to the parking area.

MARCH

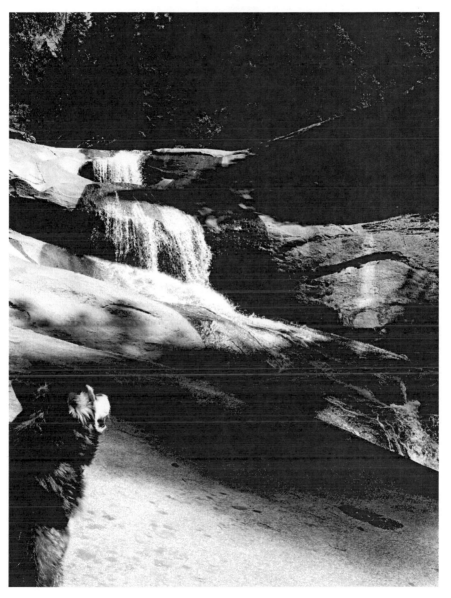

Water slide at University Falls

MARCH

If you are ready for a more challenging snowshoeing experience, then you will enjoy the one at Loon Lake. Additionally this month, you visit two waterfalls, first the more impressive University Falls, and then the falls at Bear River. At Peninsula Campground, you visit the park when the day use fees are lower as compared to the spring/summer rates. For those with physical disabilities, consider this trip, but just do the one-mile Oaks Nature Trail discovery walk.

Hike 9 - Trail to Loon Lake Chalet
Loon Lake, Crystal Basin

Difficulty: 2 (varies with snow conditions)
Distance: 1.25 miles to Chalet
Elevation: 35-foot gain from trailhead to Chalet

Directions: From Highway 50 going east, turn left onto Ice House Road immediately after crossing the bridge over the South Fork American River (about 22 miles east of Placerville). Follow Ice House Road for 24.3 miles to a right turn to Loon Lake. Proceed 4.5 miles to the road into Loon Lake Campground. In March, the campground gate is closed and you will have to park outside of the campground entrance.

Description: The whole family will enjoy this snowshoeing trail. Here you will get to test your tracking abilities to find the trail markers along the way.

From the parking area along the road, go 0.2 mile to the trailhead on your left. You should see a blue diamond marker on a tree ahead of your starting point. In addition to the diamond markers, there are numerous ribbons tied to trees to mark your way. Always look ahead to the next marker before going forward. If you look backwards, you will see the diamonds on the other side of the tree for your return trip.

After 0.5 mile, the trail crosses an asphalt service road. Look ahead in your original direction, across the road, and spot your next blue diamond marker. In another 0.1 mile, you will reach a pond and depending on the amount of water, you may need to divert around it before getting to your next marker. At 0.75 mile, you will reach a gravel service road to a power plant. The main road is immediately to your left.

Walk up to the main road and go right 0.15 mile to the Chalet. You will see the sign for the Loon Lake Chalet on your left. The Chalet provides a great picnic spot with a large deck and benches and tables (and toilet facilities). After April 1, private parties can rent the Chalet, but you should still be able to enjoy the outdoor deck. Return on your same route – easier now as you can follow your own tracks.

If you want to continue your adventure, then snowshoe down the campground road to reach Loon Lake. The Lake is beautiful this time of the year, with its frozen patches and snowy boundaries, creating silver reflections. With luck, you will visit on a sunny day, and you can make use of one of the picnic tables overlooking the lake.

Hike 10 - Darrington Trail to Salmon Falls Bridge
Peninsula Campground
Pilot Hill, CA

Difficulty: 2

Distance: Complete trail is 7.0 miles one way, so just walk as far as you want, take a break, and then turn around (you will cover the other half of the trail later in hike 15)

Elevation: 300 feet elevation change, with a few 50-foot climbs; a lot of level area also

Directions: On Highway 49 in Pilot Hill, take Rattlesnake Bar 9.0 miles to Peninsula Campground. Pay the Day Use Fee (before spring $5.00/spring & summer $8.00) at the entrance (if kiosk is not manned, then deposit envelope in green pipe at front of kiosk).

Drive in the direction of the campground to the road's end with the "Authorized Vehicles Only" gate. This is the road to the trailhead; however, there is no parking here. Drive into the campground and follow the signs to the boat launch. Here there is plenty of parking and a short trek back to the gate. Walk through the gate on the paved road a short distance. Looking ahead, you will see the green gate crossing the trail. If you are staying at the campground, you can find the Meadow Trail by walking behind campsites 85-87.

Description: You start on the Meadow Trail to Salmon Falls Bridge. The trail starts up a shaded hill and continues uphill to the left for 1.6 miles. At the crest of the hill, you will see a signpost. Continue straight here to join the Darrington Trail in the direction of Peninsula Road Crossing.

The trail winds down into view of the South Fork American River arm of Folsom Lake. There are numerous spots to go down to the lake and streams to cross, providing plenty of water and fun for your dog.

35

The trail itself is sunny, but plenty of oaks line it to provide a shady respite. Early in March, there will be less traffic on the trail, but later in March, you are likely to find more wildflowers in bloom. Watch out for the poison oak beginning to leaf out along the trail.

For the less ambitious hikers, park instead at the first parking area on the road to the campground. This area is the trailhead for a one-mile discovery walk, called The Oaks Nature Trail. There is also a small, shaded picnic area at the trailhead. This nature trail also leads you to the boat launch, so you could add this section to the overall hike if you chose.

Share with: Bikers and horses

Hike 11 - University Falls
Quintette, CA

Difficulty: 2

Distance: 2.8 miles to the falls

Elevation: 660-foot drop from trailhead to falls; otherwise, a mostly steady grade, with two 300-foot sections

Directions: From Highway 49 in Coloma/Lotus, take the Marshall Road turn in the direction of Garden Valley and Georgetown. In Georgetown, turn right onto Main Street. From Main Street, travel east out of town 11.8 miles towards Quintette (Main Street becomes Wentworth Springs Road when you leave Georgetown). Look for the yellow service gate on your left and a small parking area.

Description: This hike features a trip down to the top of University Falls on Pilot Creek. From here, you see the three water slides popular with swimmers in the summer. Hiking here in March will be less crowded, although still popular. You may also encounter snow patches, since the elevation at Quintette is 4039'. If the lower elevations received a lot of snow this winter, then save this hike for the end of March or it may become a snowshoeing adventure.

Starting through the yellow gate along the dirt service road, pass the first fork in the road (signed 12N67C) and proceed for 0.6 mile to the next fork in the road. Take the left fork labeled 12N67B. Continue along this path for another 0.9 mile to a fork at the end of a deforested area (enjoy a nice vista from here across to some distant mountains). Do not continue straight, but take the sharp right turn leading you downhill.

You will pick up a water ditch along the right hand side of the trail and hear the waters of Pilot Creek on your left. Wind down the hill another 0.9 mile, always with the ditch on your right. Look for the wide spur trail on your left. Walk in on this trail a short distance to an abandoned campsite. Looking to your right, you will see another trail. This one leads you down to Pilot Creek. This last part of the trip takes you down a gully in places, and you need to go slowly to carefully make your way down this 0.4-mile 300-foot drop. Once you reach the creek, follow it downstream to the waterfalls.

Consider a return trip here in late summer (after Labor Day weekend) to watch swimmers shoot down the three water slides. There is a fourth slide with about a 30' drop, but it is too dangerous to attempt, with a perilous climb back up. The other three slides drop about 40 feet altogether. If you cross the creek (in the summer), you may be able to walk down along the rocks bordering it and get a better view back up to the falls. Do not attempt the rocks in the spring, since they are too slippery. And never attempt the fourth slide.

Hike 12 - Bear River Campground
Trail to Bear Falls
Colfax, CA

Difficulty: 2
Distance: 2-mile loop
Elevation: 200 feet

Directions: 15.0 miles east of Auburn on I-80 in Colfax, take the Highway 174 Colfax and Grass Valley Exit, following the signs to curve around and go back over the freeway. At the Stop sign, turn right onto S. Auburn Avenue and follow it 0.3 mile until the road curves to the left, becoming Grass Valley Street. Travel on Grass Valley Street for 0.3 mile and make a left onto Rising Sun Road. Travel 0.2 mile and make a left onto Tokayana Way. Go 0.8 mile and make a right onto Milk Ranch Road

At most turns, there are signs for Bear River Campground to follow. Stay on Milk Ranch Road and you arrive at the campground entrance in 1.6 miles. Travel through the campground 0.6 mile and find the large gravel parking area on the right. The trail starts at the green gate at the far end of the parking and picnic area.

Description: If you can ignore the fact that the 20-foot falls you visit appear to come from a ditch overhead, then everyone in the family should enjoy this outing. Be sure to bring your camera for some pretty shots at the falls and perhaps your gold pans to try your luck at the river.

The trail starts on a gravel service road following along Bear River en route to the group camping area. There are plenty of access spots to stop along the river or to watch gold miners at work, some with shovels and some in full scuba gear floating in the shallow, clear waters turning over rocks. Along the way, you pass two trails taking off to the left (at

0.2 and 0.4 mile), but stay straight on the service road to the group campground (you will be returning on the loop by way of the latter trail). You will reach the campground at 0.9 mile. Here look for the second bathroom on your left and the trail that starts immediately after it. If you cross the creek in the campground, you have gone too far.

Starting now on the dirt trail, walk uphill, following Osita Creek on your right (again, do not cross the creek here). Continue 0.2 mile with a 100-foot elevation gain to Bear Falls just before the trail veers left and away from the creek. You can cross the creek at the falls (easy rock hop) and there is a trail taking you to the base with a pretty, aquamarine pool below.

For the less ambitious, turn around here and return the way you came; otherwise, continue away from the creek along the loop. You make another 100-foot elevation gain, and walk through a pleasant forest of oaks and pines, before returning down to the service road. There is a lot of poison oak along this portion of the hike, so be wary and careful to stay on the trail.

There is plenty here to enjoy at the picnic area and along the river itself. The river is peaceful, inviting you to linger here. After leaving the campground, you can stop in the old part of Colfax to shop for antiques or get an ice cream. Just turn onto Main Street from Grass Valley Street at the four-way stop.

APRIL

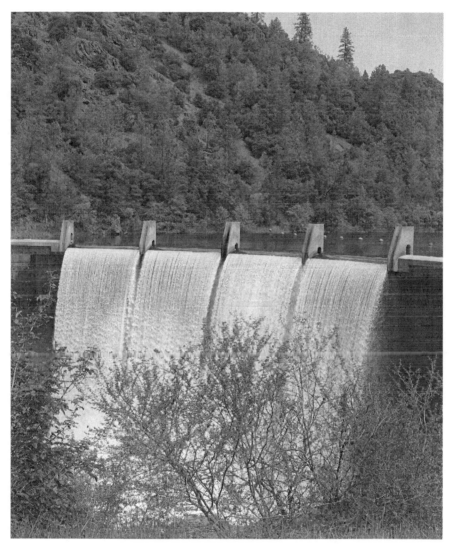

Spillway at Lake Clementine

APRIL

The wildflowers are bursting out in the foothills, so the April hikes will take you to some prime viewing spots. At Buttermilk Bend, docents have marked the trail with identifying markers for the various flowers and native brush. This is an ideal trail for those with physical limitations. On the Lake Clementine Trail, you will walk under the famous Foresthill Bridge, arriving at the end of the trail to awe over Clementine Dam's loud, cascading overflow.

Hike 13 - Buttermilk Bend
South Yuba River State Park
Bridgeport, CA

Difficulty: 1

Distance: 2.4 miles (in and out)

Elevation: 75-foot change – mostly flat trail

Warning: *Limited access for dogs May-September in park*

Directions: From Highway 49 in Grass Valley, take the Marysville exit for Highway 20 in the direction of Penn Valley and Marysville. Proceed 7.6 miles to Penn Valley and turn right onto Pleasant Valley Road. Go 7.9 miles to the South Yuba River State Park, cross the bridge, and park in the large gravel lot on the right.

Description: The Buttermilk Bend trail starts at the left end of the parking area. The trail parallels the South Fork Yuba River for its 1.2-mile length. The first half should be suitable for those with walkers. You should plan on leashing and scooping for your dog on this very popular trail. At the peak of wildflower season, it can be crowded.

Along the way, you will find numerous wildflowers and native brush with labeled markers for easy identification. There are many picture-taking opportunities of the flowers and the beautiful river below. Be on the lookout for flowers without labels, such as a display of petite red maids at the start of the trail.

In addition, numerous spur trails offer a path down to the river for a break and a splash for your dog. The trail itself has a number of benches for stops and a bridge crossing a nice creek with access to it above the bridge. If you use a walker, then the bridge will be your turn around point.

This trail could easily accommodate those with physical limitations, so everyone in the family can enjoy this outing. At times, there are steep drop-offs, so if you are afraid of precipices you may want to reconsider taking this hike.

Notes: Celebrate **Living History Day** at the park on the last Sunday of April. There are period costumes, covered buggy rides, panning demonstrations, and much more for learning about the history of the area. Phone the park at (530) 432-2546 to verify the date and time for the event.

Hike 14 - Quarry Road Trail
Auburn State Recreation Area
Middle Fork American River

Difficulty: First 1.25 miles level, a 1 difficulty;
remaining miles a 2 difficulty

Distance: 5.6 miles one-way (you can shorten)

Elevation: 270 feet overall gain, with several 50-
100 foot "ups and downs"

Directions: On Highway 49 between Cool and Auburn, 0.25 mile south of the American River crossing at Old Foresthill Road, you will find the parking area for Quarry Road Trail on the river's side of the highway. The trailhead is at the far end of the parking area.

Description: This is a scenic walk in the canyon of the Middle Fork American River. You start upstream on a wide, flat trail for the first 1.25 miles, so even those with physical limitations should be able to enjoy this part. Tricycles, strollers, and walkers will work on the first part of the trail. Two spots (at 0.2 and 0.6 mile) have picnic tables, and then at the 1.25 mark there is a large picnic area. For the less ambitious, or families with small children, plan to do this part of the walk and then return to your car. Children will have fun watching geese and ducks sunning on rocks or leisurely floating, and finding spots to scramble down to the water.

For the more adventurous hikers, continue from the picnic area, bearing right up the trail going uphill. Here, you will pass by remains of an old limestone-loading platform, a tunnel, and a cave welcoming you for a peek inside. The trail leaves the river canyon as you cross by a number of streams flowing into the river. At the 2.0-mile mark, you will intersect with the Western States Trail, where you will continue in the direction of Brown's Bar Trail, with the trail returning closer to the river.

Soon you will begin to hear the sounds coming from the off-road vehicles at the Mammoth Bar Off-Highway Vehicle (OHV) Park across the river. You can pause on your side of the river and watch the bikes traversing the dirt paths up the canyon walls. The sound will carry with you along the trail for a while, but it is dim enough so as not to be an annoyance.

Foothill brush, oaks, madrones, olive trees, buckeyes, and digger pines line the trail. Beware the blackberry vines and poison oak plants along the sides. It is a well-maintained trail, so as long as you avoid going off-trail, you should not have any problems.

At 2.75 miles, the trail descends close to the river's edge, making for easy access to its bank. This is a nice resting place (and possible turnaround). Continuing on, at 3.5 miles, you reach the Brown's Bar Trail. Stay on the Western States Trail in the direction of Maine Bar Trail. At 4.5 miles, again the trail touches down to river level. Although you will have to cross a field of river rocks to reach its edge, you have easy access to a nice deep, clear, pool of calm water. This is again a possible turnaround point or you can continue on the trail, now narrower, another mile to the intersection with the Maine Bar Trail, before ending at Maine Bar at 5.6 miles.

The scenery is beautiful on this very popular trail. You will encounter bikers, joggers, horseback riders, and families throughout your day. It is best to come earlier in the day to avoid the larger crowds.

Notes: Mammoth Bar OHV Park, part of the Auburn State Recreation Area, has no fees and is open year round (canyon trails closed on Saturdays). It features 1200 acres, combining scenic steep canyon and river rides on well-marked and maintained trails. A beginner's loop is available as well.

Hike 15 - Darrington Mountain Bike Trail
El Dorado Hills, CA

Difficulty: 2

Distance: Varies

Elevation: About 40 total feet up and down from trailhead with mostly a flat trail involving occasional 20-foot "ups and downs"

Directions: When El Dorado Hills Boulevard crosses Green Valley Road, it becomes Salmon Falls Road. Go 5.7 miles on Salmon Falls Road in the direction of Pilot Hill. You park in the gravel area on your left, just before reaching the Salmon Falls Bridge. Walk 0.16 mile across the bridge and past Skunk Hollow to the trailhead parking on your left.

Both the trailhead parking and the Skunk Hollow parking are fee, self-registration parking areas, so parking on the other side of the bridge saves you money.

Description: Bring a picnic blanket for this beautiful, easy hike. At a little short of 3.0 miles, there is a lovely open area to sit, looking out to the lake. Along the way, you cross several streams and plenty of access spots to the water for your dog. Wildflowers are starting to come out now for your enjoyment. There is no real destination, just walk for as long as you want and then turn around for the hike back to your car.

The trail starts with a short 20-foot climb before leveling out. When you reach the "Y", either choice will bring you to the same place in a short distance. The narrow, rocky, dirt trail parallels the South Fork American River. Then you will drop down to a small stream where the trail widens for awhile, taking you by fields of lupine.

Within 45 minutes, you will be at another stream crossing. Your trail is lined first with oaks and then with native brush. At 2.5 miles, there is another "Y" and again either route takes you to the same place (the left arm looks much easier). If you go beyond 3.0 miles, your elevation will rise a little.

The entire length of the trail is over 7.0 miles, so plan to hike whatever portion is comfortable and fits your time schedule. If you did the Peninsula Campground hike, then you already did the other half of the trail.

Share with: Bikers

Hike 16 - Lake Clementine Trail
North Fork American River
Auburn, CA

Difficulty: 2
Distance: 4.0 miles roundtrip
Elevation: 365 feet

Before the hike: Stop at **Coloma Club Café** at 7171 Highway 49 (at Marshall Road) for a fine home-style breakfast. (Seasonal dog-friendly outdoor dining) (530) 626-6390

Directions: At the junction of Highway 49 and Old Foresthill Road south of Auburn, take Old Foresthill Road about 0.25 miles and cross the Old Foresthill Bridge. Immediately after crossing the bridge, the trailhead is at the green gate on your left, marked with the number 139. Parking is available on either side of the road.

Description: This 2.0-mile trail takes you upstream along the North Fork American River, featuring a walk under the new Foresthill Bridge and culminating at the spillway for Lake Clementine. Along the way are marked posts 5-10 pointing out spots of interest. For detailed descriptions, and historical background, contact the Auburn State Recreation Area for their self-guided pamphlet (530-885-4527).

The trail starts out level with Marker #5 at the beginning, inviting you to gaze at the Foresthill Bridge ahead. Built originally to accommodate the lake generated by the now abandoned Auburn Dam project, the bridge is now the tallest one in California at 730 feet. Marker #6 points to the lack of larger trees in the area due to many fires in the area. At Marker #7, you see the remaining concrete abutments for the old steel bridge, which stood there from 1911-1955. Marker #8 again points to the new bridge and a closer look at its concrete abutments. Marker #9 designates the beginnings of Clarks Hole, a section of still water along the river popular for swimming in the summer, and for year round fishing. A bar in the river of raised sand and boulders forms the hole. There is an easy access trail down to the river here and a nice beach also.

At the last post, Marker #10, you look across the river to see the remains of an old covered wooden bridge in service from 1875-1911. The bridge served to collect tolls for travelers between Foresthill and Auburn. For the less-ambitious hikers, this will be your perfect turnaround point.

Continuing beyond the last marker, the trail steadily climbs along a wide dirt service road. At about the 1-mile point, there is a spur trail to a nice fishing spot (150-foot drop from main trail to river). After another 0.25 mile, you can hear the flow from Lake Clementine ahead and peek through the trees to see the spillway waters in the distance. At 1.6 miles, you exit the trail through the green gate and walk to the road. Bear a sharp left into the park and continue down this road about 0.3 miles to a spur trail on your left taking you to the spillway. Here you will have a great view of Lake Clementine and the North Fork Dam, the cascading water and its cool spray.

Share with: Bikers

MAY

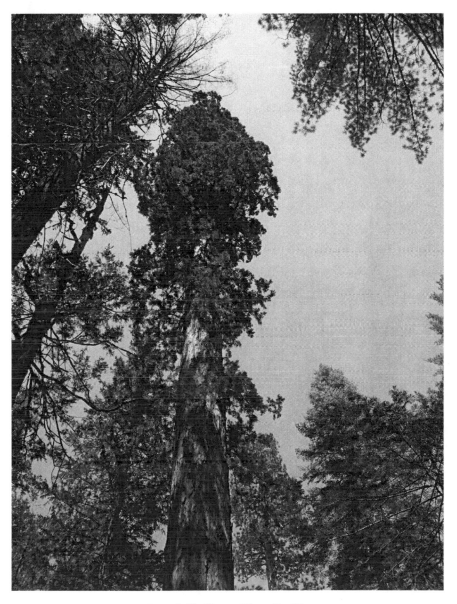

Giant Joffre Tree at Placer Big Trees

MAY

This month's hikes continue to seek wildflowers with the Olmstead Loop Trail, Dave Moore Nature Area, and Independence Trail. Both the Dave Moore Nature Area and Independence Trail offer access to those with physical limitations. The other May hike takes you to the Placer Big Trees Grove to view some of the largest trees in the area. This hike is also an interpretive trail, making for a great multi-generational family experience.

Hike 17 - The Placer Big Trees Grove
Tahoe National Forest
Foresthill, CA

Difficulty: 1

Distance: 2.5 miles with two intersecting loops

Elevation: 200 feet gain

Directions: From I-80 in Auburn, take the Foresthill exit to Foresthill Road. Drive 15.5 miles to Foresthill and the U.S. Forest Service Foresthill Ranger Station. Pick up a pamphlet there for The Placer Big Trees Grove. When they are not open, their outdoor information kiosk should have some pamphlets for you. You can call ahead to (530) 367-2224 for more information.

From the Ranger Station, continue on Foresthill Road 1.2 miles and turn right onto Mosquito Ridge Road. Drive just beyond the 24-mile marker, and find on your right the turn marked for the Placer Big Trees. Then make an immediate right turn, following the sign to the Big Trees parking area 0.5 mile down the road. At the upper parking area, there are picnic tables, restrooms, water, and barbeques.

Description: Rev up the Ferrari or your Harley for this trip. While this is a long drive for a short walk, the drive itself on Mosquito Ridge Road is rewarding, with views of deep canyons and the distant snow-capped Sierra Nevada mountains. It is a windy road, and you have to take your time traversing it. The reward is a walk through the northernmost grove of Giant Sequoias. Also in this old growth forest, you will find Ponderosa and Sugar Pines, giant Douglas firs, and a 250-foot Joffre tree. It is an easy enough hike the entire family can enjoy (not recommended for the less ambulatory). Along the way, there are 17 posts marking points of interest. The pamphlet you picked up at the Ranger Station will detail what you can see at each post, helping you through this self-guided interpretive trail.

There are two intersecting loops at the grove. One is the Forest View Trail, which has starting points from the parking area or at Marker #13 in the Big Trees Loop. The Forest View Trail is 1.0 mile in length, taking you through the old growth forest. The Big Trees Loop is the interpretive trail explaining the history and the science of the many giant trees. The problem is that the two trails intersect in the middle of the Big Trees Loop, causing you to either skip part of the Big Trees Loop (not recommended), or having to repeat half of the Big Trees Loop (better choice) in order to do both.

Start with the Big Trees Loop and walk from markers 1 to 13. At Marker #13, you will see the sign for the Forest View Trail to the right. Start the view trail here and wind your way through the forest. You will end back at the parking lot. Then start the Big Trees Loop again, repeating markers 1 to13, and then continuing the loop for the remaining markers 14 to17. For the less ambitious, just do the Big Trees Loop and forget about the Forest View Trail.

Notes: If you do not acquire a pamphlet, you can use the following as a guide.

(1)   Observe the different trees and shrubs in the grove.

(2)   Feel the bark of the Ponderosa Pine.

(3)   See a decomposing tree.

(4)   Site the 500-year old Douglas fir tree.

(5)   Enjoy the Giant Sequoia.

(6)   Look for a Western Azalea in bloom.

(7)   Note the foliage of these younger Giant Sequoias.

(8)   See a Giant Sequoia that fell in 1861.

(9)   See algae growing on the Giant Sequoia and the hollow resulting from a fire.

(10) Listen for water draining underground.

(11) Visit the base of the Roosevelt Tree, another fallen Giant Sequoia.

(12) Gaze up at the tallest tree in the grove, the Joffre tree over 250 feet tall.

(13) View here the Pershing Tree, the largest tree by volume in the grove.

(14) Again, you are at the Roosevelt Tree.

(15) View a rotting fir.

(16) Notice the growth of the cedar before you to support the fallen cedar next to it.

(17) See the holes caused by woodpeckers and insects.

The pamphlet best explains how fires and storms have affected this grove, and how natural decomposition and underground water nourish the survivors.

Hike 18 - Olmstead Loop (Knickerbocker Trail) Cool, CA

Difficulty: 2

Distance: 7.9-mile loop

Elevation: Rolling trail with two steep ascents of 130 feet and 270 feet

Warnings: *Share the trail with mountain bikers and equestrians – always yield to equestrians. My dog likes going off-trail and we found at least 100 ticks on her last May after this hike.*

Directions: On Highway 49 in Cool turn on Saint Florian Court at the fire station and find the parking area just behind it. The first level of parking is for cars, and the upper level is for horse trailers. If you are coming from Auburn, it is a right turn on St. Florian Court just before the fire station and the Stop sign. Coming from Coloma, make a left turn just after the Stop sign in Cool and the fire station.

Description: This is a fun hike with lots of wildflowers and wildlife to see, along with vernal pools and a couple of creek crossings. Additionally, great views across the American River Canyon and the foothills will award you.

You are going to do this loop in reverse of the marked order (so you will start at the 9.0-mile marker instead of in the 0.0 direction). You will be going in a counter-clockwise direction. Going in the prescribed clockwise direction, I always get lost due to the pond covering the trail in the first mile. Starting in the reverse direction, you cross Saint Florian Court and pick up the trail on the other side of the road.

At first, you will parallel Highway 49, but in 0.25 mile, you will turn away from its traffic and start to enjoy the rolling hills with 50-foot "ups and downs", passing the marker for Quarry Trail to the right. In less than 0.5 mile, the Olmstead Loop veers to the right (you will see the trail marker on its path). You will stay straight here, making a little shortcut. For the next 0.5 mile, continue along this shortcut, taking in the tree-lined trail of oaks, passing an old shack and a pond, and then rejoining the loop. Turn left here to continue the loop.

Now you will pass by some rock outcroppings on your left and then come to the 6.5-mile marker for the trail. Soon the trail curves to your right and starts descending to Salt Creek (avoid the narrow spur trails, staying on the wider actual trail). Along the way down, you will come to a nice water spot for your dog. If you look to the left, you will see a pond also. The pond can be a little murky, but my dog likes running in it nevertheless. Continuing on, you reach Salt Creek (not impressive). From the creek crossing, it is a 270-foot ascent, passing by a trail on the right signed Coffer Dam Trail (which takes you down to the diversion tunnel).

As you continue along the loop, you will see remnants of ranches that existed before the government took the land for public use for the Auburn Dam Project. The U.S. Bureau of Reclamation now owns the land and the California Park System administers it. The trail was formerly called the Knickerbocker Trail before Dan Olmstead organized bikers to establish a trail to be enjoyed by hikers, bikers, and equestrians together.

Enjoy the rolling hills and the views across the canyon. You will descend once more, down to Knickerbocker Creek. This is a good resting spot, with a loud flow of water, and pools to splash in. After your rest, there is a 130-foot ascent through a pine forest. You will find mile markers at every 0.5 mile and the trail is easy to follow (avoid spurs and stay on the dirt road) until the last mile when the trail marker leads you left into a marsh. You need to stay straight instead to go around the water. You will find a bridge to your left to help you cross over the water. Looking ahead, you will again see the trail and be able to follow it back to the parking area.

Be sure to bring a camera, because you will see a variety of wildflowers on this hike. Look for the illusive Red Maid that only opens on a sunny day. Bring your wildflower book to help with identifying the various species here.

Now that you know the trail's nuances, the next time you visit here you can do the hike in the prescribed clockwise direction, starting at mile 0.0. You should be able to bypass the path into the pond successfully, and make your way around the loop following the trail markers. Look for the marker for the short cut, or else you will add another mile to the loop. Going in this direction, the ascents from the Knickerbocker and Salt Creek are much easier.

Less Ambitious Option: Try the trail in its clockwise direction and get lost just as I do after a mile when you reach the marsh. You will see a trail along the right of the marsh that will meander a bit and take you back to the parking area. You will still see a variety of wildflowers and be able to enjoy the scenery doing this shorter hike.

Share with: Bikers and horses

Hike 19 - Dave Moore Nature Area
South Fork American River
Lotus, CA

Difficulty: 1
Distance: 1.0 mile loop trail (including spur trails)
Elevation: 80-foot change in elevation

Before the hike: Stop at **Sierra Rizing Bakery** to pick up
some treats or maybe a bread loaf for tonight's
dinner. The bakery is immediately across the
bridge on the left in Lotus. (530) 642-1308

Directions: For detailed directions to the intersection of Lotus Road
and Highway 49, see Hike 1. When Lotus Road dead ends at Highway
49, turn left and cross the bridge over the South Fork American River.
In 1.0 mile after crossing the bridge, you will see the rock wall entrance
for the Dave Moore Nature Area on your left. (Before April 1ˢᵗ the
entrance gate is closed, so park outside the park and walk down to the
trailhead.)

Coming from the other direction, from I-80 in Auburn, connect
with Highway 49 south towards Cool. The entrance to the nature
area will be on your right about 3.0 miles south of Pilot Hill. From
Placerville, take Highway 49 through Coloma. At the three-way stop
at Lotus Road and Highway 49, continue straight across the bridge.
Go 1.0 mile after the bridge to find the entrance on the left.

Description: This is an easy hike, maintained by the Bureau of Land
Management (BLM). The trail features many picnic tables and access
to the American River. Most importantly, the first part of the hike
is accessible to anyone physically challenged. A monument with a
plaque is located at the start of your walk honoring Dave Moore, a

BLM employee afflicted with multiple sclerosis at the age of 35. His co-workers and other volunteers worked together to create a nature area that all could enjoy.

Start the hike from the parking area in a counter-clockwise direction. After passing numerous streams and some picnic tables (two specifically designed for wheelchair access), you will come to an interesting rock at 0.2 mile. The rock's composition is such that its center eroded more quickly (from wind and other elements), forming a mushroom-like appearance.

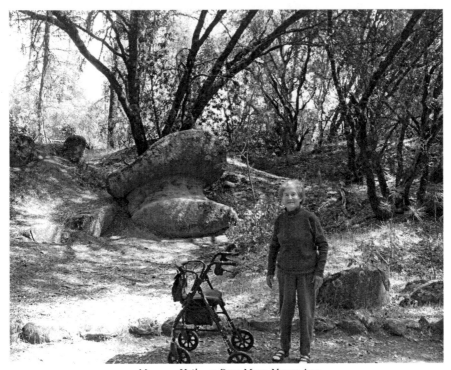

My mom, Hailey, at Dave Moore Nature Area

The trail then turns into an area with large ponderosa pines with their "patchwork" bark, their needles blanketing your walk. At 0.26 mile, you will come to a grand madrone tree with its beautiful reddish bark. Round the bend to find a rock wall lining the way and listen for the river ahead. It is just a few minutes now to the spur trail taking you down to the South Fork American River.

Pause here at the river and enjoy its peacefulness. In the coming months, there will be a constant stream of rafts and kayakers maneuvering their way down the river's rocky lanes. Another beach awaits you, so return to the main trail to continue the loop. (For the physically challenged, this is the turnaround spot, since the trail will now narrow and is uneven and rocky for a while.)

In less than 0.1 mile, you will see a large boulder bordering the left side of the trail. Just before the rock, a spur trail takes off to your right, returning you to the river and a nice beach with beautiful black sand beckoning you to gold panning. If this beach is occupied, continue along the beach upstream to an equally nice alternative.

Leaving the river, the trail again becomes even and easy to navigate. It is dotted with beautiful rock formations. Some spurs exist, but stay on the main trail (the BLM have marked off the spurs with branches and burlap rolls to indicate they are closed). Start a short ascent now, with the trail lined with manzanita shrubs. After the climb, you will head back through a grove of oaks, cross a bridge, and return to the parking area. Just across the bridge (before the parking area), there is a picnic area up the hill.

For the physically challenged having to turn around at the river and not complete the loop, cross the bridge at the other end of the loop and go 200 feet in a clockwise direction. This will take you to a wonderful spot for wildflowers, with baby blue-eyes, five spots (early bloomers), and many more to enjoy and photograph. You can continue in this direction for a while before needing to turn around again.

You can return to the nature area in the coming weeks to find a constant display of new wildflowers emerging weekly, such as pretty face, California poppies, globe lilies, and lacepod. On your revisit, do the loop in the reverse direction and you will definitely see new parts and angles of the trail to photograph or sketch. Return throughout the year to experience the different seasons and enjoy the river at different water levels. Things change constantly here, and every time you visit, you are sure to see something new.

Hike 20 - Independence Trail
Nevada City, CA

Difficulty: 1
Distance: Varies
Elevation: Flat trail; wheelchair accessible

Directions: Where Highways 49 and 20 split in Nevada City, you will take a left turn and stay on 49 in the direction of Downieville. Travel 6.4 miles on Highway 49 to the signed Independence Trail with plenty of parking along the shoulder of the highway.

Description: This is a wheelchair accessible, flat trail, great for small children and those with physical limitations. There are two trail options, the West and the East trails. They do not intersect and both are in and out walks. The West goes 2.6 miles and the East another 2.2 miles, so you can opt to do one of these, both, or portions of either one.

The trail is nicely shaded and in spring full of wildflowers. The trail docents have marked many of the flowers and native bushes and trees with their scientific and common names. The trail has many points of interest and historical influences. On the West trail, there is an overlook with a fantastic view down to the South Fork Yuba River.

There are reconstructed flumes originally used by miners for hydraulic mining, as well as benches and picnic tables for relaxing. At the 1.0-mile mark, you can take a 0.1-mile walk down a zigzag wooden walkway to Rush Creek and view a small waterfall.

Continuing on the West route, you reach Flume 32 and Jones Ravine at the 2.6-mile point. The East trail also offers flumes and takes you to the Miners Tunnel Overlook at the 2.2-mile point.

Everyone in the family should enjoy this outing, especially the flower enthusiast. After enjoying Independence Trail, you can continue your day with a stroll through the streets of Nevada City.

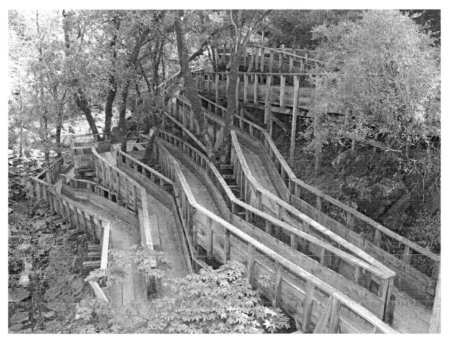

Zigzag walkway to Rush Creek

JUNE

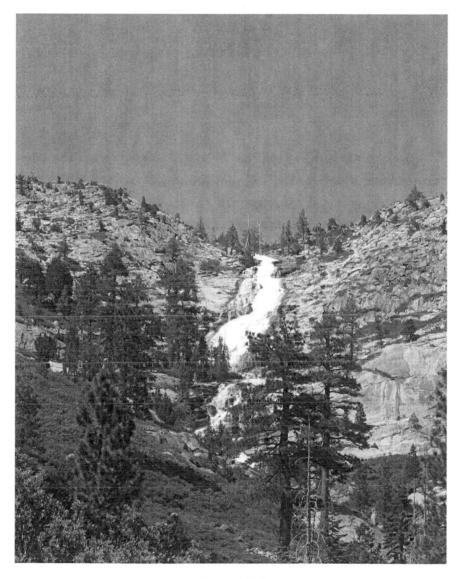

Horsetail Falls

JUNE

With luck, this month you can start hitting the higher elevations unless there was late snowfall. You will start the month in the foothills with an easy walk around the Georgetown Nature Area. While easy, it can be slippery with the pine needles for those with balance issues. If you have physical limitations, then you definitely want to do the hike at the Tallac Historic Site and visit the Taylor Creek Visitor Center. For the most adventurous, you have the hike to Horsetail Falls. The Caples Creek hike is one of my favorites, with rewarding meadows, rock formations, and the noisy cascades from the creek.

Hike 21 - Georgetown Nature Area
Georgetown, CA

Difficulty: 1

Distance: 1.0-3.0 miles depending on selected trails

Elevation: 100 foot gain/loss from trailhead

Directions: From Main Street in Georgetown, turn right onto Harkness Street (0.2 mile to second right). Go 0.3 mile on Harkness Street to the parking area for the Georgetown Nature Area on your left adjacent to Georgetown School.

Description: The Georgetown Nature Area is a fenced park covering 35 acres. Within the park, numerous trails (mostly well-marked and labeled) crisscross throughout, taking you over streams to an old gold mine, a native plants area, a big trees forest, and an Indian exhibit. You visit ponds where you can easily spot fish and frogs, and a meadow. Markers name many of the trees throughout the area.

You start at the South entrance to the park. There is an information kiosk there where you may be able to pick up a map. If you do not want to take a chance with the kiosk being stocked, you can call the Black Oak Mine Unified School District office at (530) 333-8300 before going. The map is very useful. Following the map, you can choose to walk around the park's perimeter (about 1.5 mile loop), or instead choose to visit specific points of interest. The most direct route to the old gold mine and the Indian Village is 0.5 mile.

If you are unlucky in acquiring a map, let me suggest the following route. Shortly after going through the entrance, take the first trail to the right, called Big Trees Trail. Along this trail, you will first pass by an old burn area, then walk through a forest of large pines and black oaks, and finally emerge at Schaeffer Meadows. From the meadows, locate the Big Foot Trail that takes you to the old gold mine. You can walk across the bridge to look inside of the mine. Then return to the other side of the creek and continue north on Rosery Hill Trail.

Stay straight on Rosery Hill (avoid the turn onto Ponderosa) to arrive at the replica Indian cedar huts. Walk around the back of the huts to the series of ponds. Cross to the other side of the ponds where the benches are located. (If you do not cross, you will walk out of the park at its North Entrance.) From the ponds, walk to the backside of the huts and find Alder Creek Trail. This trail will take you to a long wooden bridge. Before reaching the end of this bridge, take the Oak Canyon Trail to the right.

On the Oak Canyon Trail, you will walk by the Native Plants site. Some of the plants have labels for you, while other labels may be missing. After the Native Plants area, take a right onto Manzanita Trail. Then take a left onto Orchard Trail to take you back to the South Entrance. If you miss the turn onto Orchard (not hard to do), you may find yourself walking out of the West gate at the amphitheatre. If this happens, come back into the park and make the first possible right, again looking for the marker to Orchard Trail.

Even with a map, traversing the area is a little tricky. However, you should be able to easily retrace your steps and find the South gate. Otherwise, you can go out to the road from the amphitheatre and walk down to the parking area.

After the hike: Park on Main Street in Georgetown and walk along the businesses. From Main Street, if you walk down Highway 193 (right from Main Street), you can visit the Pioneer Cemetery officially opened in 1852, but with a marker dating back to 1850. You may also have noticed the old Ten Stamp Mill at the corner of Harkness and Main on your way to the Nature Area. You are bound to see some interesting people in downtown Georgetown while you enjoy walking its Main Street with cars parked in the center of the road.

Hike 22 - Tallac Historic Site and Taylor Creek Visitor Center Camp Richardson, CA

Difficulty: 1

Distance: 5-mile round trip

Elevation: This is a flat walk with a 15-foot change in elevation overall

Directions: At the 'Y' in South Lake Tahoe on Highway 50, continue straight on Highway 89 in the direction of Tahoe City. Go 1.4 miles and park on the right shoulder near Marker #46). The bike trail is a little further in from the road on the right. Start on the bike trail going left in the direction of Camp Richardson and Tahoe City.

Description: This is an enjoyable walk, at times on a bike trail, and at others on an unpaved walking trail. You visit the Tallac Historic Site with refurbished old estates to tour, gardens to stroll, and weekend festivities to enjoy. In 2007, a sampling of events included a Celtic Festival, a Quilt Show, and a Tibetan Festival. You can check www.valhallatahoe. com, or phone (530) 541-5227, to see what the scheduled activities are for the day you plan to visit. You also walk to the Taylor Creek Visitor Center with a 0.5-mile loop Rainbow Trail and an underground stream chamber for viewing underwater wildlife.

Starting on the paved bike trail, after 0.2 mile, you will find a spur trail leading away towards the lake. You can take this to a wildlife sanctuary, a marsh, and a view of Tahoe Keys. At Pope Beach (no dogs allowed at Pope Beach), you need to return to the bike trail to reach Camp Richardson. In town, there are numerous stores and eateries, as well as a trolley car. Continue on the bike trail through the town until you see the sign directing you to the Tallac Historic Site to the right. Take this paved trail to reach the park.

At the Tallac Historic Site, you can stroll past three refurbished estates: Valhalla, Pope, and Baldwin. At the Baldwin Estate, you can get maps and information and purchase tickets for touring the Pope Estate. Also on the grounds are the servants quarters furnished in the style of the early 1900's. You can also look into the old dairy, guest cottages, and kitchen.

Two old boathouses remain (now theatres), along with a barn, and garage. From the boathouses, you can access the beach (dogs allowed). Numerous benches and picnic tables are available on the grounds, as well as an arboretum and pond, and a native plants garden. Throughout the summer, starting Memorial Day weekend, they offer numerous activities, for both children and adults.

Continuing in the same direction, from Tallac, you can pick up the Tallac Historic Site Trail from the Tallac parking area (this is not the same parking area you passed on your way into the park; it is on the opposite side of the park). Walk about 15 minutes away from the lake towards the bike trail to reach the Taylor Creek Visitor Center.

At the Visitor Center, you can purchase books, maps, and postcards. There is a short Smokey's Trail for children to learn about fire safety. You can also find staff to answer any questions, and perhaps join a naturalist walk. From the Visitor Center, pick up the Rainbow Trail for a self-guided walk on this signed trail. The Rainbow Trail visits the underground stream chamber. From the chamber, you can take a short trail back to the paved bike trail and the return walk to your car.

If you return to the Taylor Creek Visitor Center in October, you can see salmon and trout spawning.

Less Ambitious Option: For those with physical limitations, you can park at both the Tallac Historic Site and the Taylor Creek Visitor Center (Marker #48 on Highway 89) and enjoy touring both. This will eliminate the walk along the bike trail, and most of the mileage.

Hike 23 - Caples Creek Trail
Kyburz, CA

Difficulty: 2

Distance: 7.75 miles roundtrip (two hours to end of trail)

Elevation: This is an uphill hike, gaining 730 feet,
including a 225-foot ascent

Directions: On Highway 50 in Kyburz, look for the "Silverfork Road 1 Mile" sign. Turn right onto Silverfork Road and proceed 9.0 miles to the trailhead on your left (0.5 mile past Silver Fork Campground). If you cross the bridge over the Silver Fork of the American River, then you have just passed the trailhead. There is plenty of parking here. At 5000' elevation, you can get to this trail in June unless it has been a heavy or late snow year. To verify Silverfork Road is open, call the Placerville Ranger Station at (530) 644-2324 (or visit www.fs.fed. us/r5/eldorado).

Description: Start up the dirt road from the parking area to reach the trailhead marked as 17E51. Within 10 minutes of this hike, you will reach Caples Creek and a great view of its cascades down rocky steps. Here you will find a post directing you left to the trail up the hill. In another 20 minutes, you will reach a beautiful waterfall.

Within 40 minutes, the waters calm and pool, enhancing some beach areas along the creek for resting or picnicking. Within one hour, you are at the first of four meadows. For the less ambitious, there are plenty of options for stopping and for the rest, continue to the destination of Government Meadows, making for a 7.75-mile round trip adventure.

In June, you may encounter a lot of water on the trail, especially through the meadows (unless it was a light rain year). You will see bright red cactus-like succulent snow plants along the creek, along with

71

creek side alders. The trail is forested with large cedar, aspen, and Jeffrey pines, and an occasional oak with its fresh new leaves. Throughout the hike, you will be treated to stunning rock formations. When you enter the second meadow, look to your left to see an impressive crag above you. The third meadow is signed as Jake Schnieder meadow.

Continue straight through this meadow towards Hay Flat and come to a final post indicating Government Meadows to your right. Turn here to find the fourth (and least impressive) meadow. Continue past the meadow another 0.25 mile to the trail's end at the creek and find a nice lunch spot. While there is loop trail available, it is difficult to follow and involves two water crossings, so I suggest you return on the same trail.

If you revisit here in October, you will enjoy a display of fall colors. If you are adventuresome, you can find the trail to the bridge across Caples Creek and a splendid view of its waters. This is a good family hike, not too difficult, and a lot of variety in terrain and ecosystems to enjoy.

Share with: Horses and two-wheeled vehicles

Hike 24 - Horsetail Falls
Pyramid Creek Trail
Twin Bridges, CA

Difficulty: 2
Distance: 3.0 miles in and out
Elevation: 760 feet gain

Directions: From Highway 50 East, about 11 miles beyond Kyburz in Twin Bridges, find the parking area for Pyramid Creek on your left. There is a center turn lane here just after a passing lane and just prior to the bridge crossing Pyramid Creek. There is a parking fee ($3.00 in 2007).

Description: Once you make it to the base of Horsetail Falls, you will never again be tempted to stop at Bridal Veil Falls on your way up to Tahoe. The falls are beautiful, loud, and photographic. The trail, however, is difficult to follow, poorly marked, and not maintained, probably due to deaths of people trying to go beyond the foot of the falls and climbing the slippery rocks to the top. You will not get lost, because on the hike up you can both see and hear the falls to give you direction. Coming back down, whatever path you take should take you back to Highway 50. Nevertheless, the hike is a tracking challenge and you may need to be happy with however far you make it.

Ideally, you want to go as soon as the snow melts, the paths and rocks have dried, and the streams lowered – you want optimum water volume with the falls, with as little water on the trail as possible. Generally, this is a great hike for June.

From the parking area, be sure to pay the day use fee before starting out on the trail. Within minutes, you will be at Pyramid Creek where the trail veers to the left, keeping the creek on your right. Continue along the creek until you reach a trail sign pointing you to the left. The trail returns to follow the creek most of the way, always with the creek on your right. A multitude of misleading spur trails abounds to steer you to the creek, but remember your goal is to go uphill to the falls.

Follow the trail posts pointing in the direction of the Wilderness Boundary. After about 0.5 mile, the trail ends at the base of a large rock slab. You must hike directly up the granite wall to rejoin the actual trail. When your climb finally plateaus, you will get your first view of the falls in the distance. If you turn around, you will have a great view of Lover's Leap looking back towards Highway 50.

After about 0.75 mile, you will enter Desolation Wilderness. There is a kiosk towards the left with day use permits to fill out. The trail continues directly from the kiosk on the right of the sign. The trail takes you along a cool creek and welcoming shade. You may have to get your feet a little wet in a heavy rainy season; otherwise, the crossings will be relatively easy. You will come to one area where you walk along a ledge skirting a small pond – yes, this is the trail. Later the trail takes you seemingly under a large rock.

You then walk up rocks towards the falls. At the last part, you hike up a gully to the trail's end at the base of the falls. Do not attempt to go any further than this; and, keep dogs away from the steep trail edges. It is too easy to slip on the flat rocks to approach the edges. The gully is safely away from the edge, but the rocks are still slippery and you can easily end up on your bottom. Use your hands to hold on to other rocks and ensure your balance.

Making it to the base is rewarding and worth any mental or physical struggles. On your way down, do not be surprised if you cannot follow the exact way you came up! This hike is definitely a challenge, but the distance is not great, the climb not too difficult, and the rewarding end well worth it.

JULY

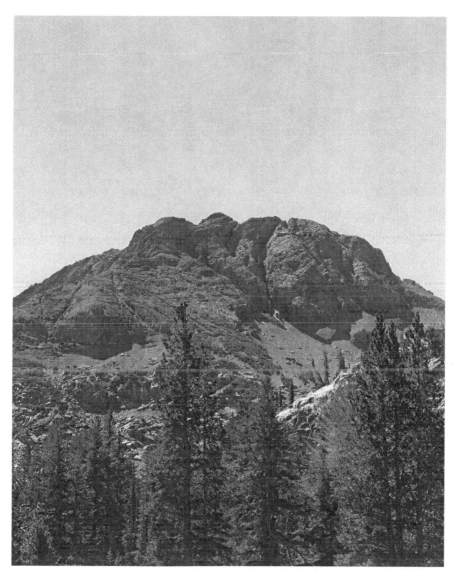

View of Round Top from Woods Lake Trail

JULY

This month you will reach two more waterfalls and visit both the Desolation and Mokelumne Wildernesses, taking the first level '3' hikes. The great part of going to the mountains for these hikes, besides escaping the valley heat, is the lack of poison oak and rattlesnakes at this higher elevation.

On the hike to Round Top Lake, you should see a great display of alpine wildflowers. The hike to Maud Lake is one of my favorites, although a bit more strenuous. All of these hikes have rewarding destinations of alpine lakes or waterfalls. If you are looking for an easy outing, then definitely go to Bassi Falls.

The wilderness trails you share with horses, mountain goats, and llamas. Always yield to these pack animals.

Hike 25 - Bassi Falls
Crystal Basin Recreation Area
Ice House Road

Difficulty: 1

Distance: 0.5 mile in to falls

Elevation: This is an easy, short hike with a little uphill of about 100 feet

Directions: From Highway 50 East, about 5.0 miles past Fresh Pond, take the left turn onto Ice House Road to the Crystal Basin Recreation Area. Drive 16.4 miles just across the bridge for Big Silver Creek and opposite the Big Silver Creek Campground, making a right onto Road 12N32A.

The road quickly becomes graded gravel and at 0.2 mile, you need to make a left turn onto the road to Bassi Falls. It is now another 1.4 miles to the parking area and trailhead, the road changing to dirt about midway, making for a dusty, bumpy ride. There is little parking (about six vehicles), and the turnaround is small, so if possible try this hike mid-week. It is short enough that you can leave work a little early and still have plenty of time to enjoy the hike.

Description: Starting from the parking area, choose the trail on the left heading uphill. You have a steady little climb through a forest of oaks, manzanita, pines, and cedars, arriving at a plateau and rock slab to cross. You should easily see the dirt trail that continues past the rocks. Follow the trail down to the falls, making a note of the trail's entrance for your return trip.

In a low rain year, the falls will not be as spectacular, but you can enjoy exploring the rocks downstream and find nice water holes. Imagine the water that must run down these polished slabs in a heavy rainy season. In a good rain year, plan your visit as soon as the roads are navigable to enjoy the falls at their peak. You may need a 4-wheel drive or high clearance vehicle in more intense rain seasons, so use good judgment. This is definitely a place you will want to go to over again, especially in years when the falls will be at their fullest.

Hike 26 - Umpa Lake
Wrights Lake Recreation Area

Difficulty: 3
Distance: 2.5 miles to the lake
Elevation: 470-foot gain before 200 feet drop down to lake

Directions: From Highway 50 East at Kyburz, continue another 4.8 miles to a left turn onto Wrights Road. Follow this road 8.1 miles into the Wrights Lake Campground. At the Stop sign, continue straight another 0.3 mile to the parking for Rockbound Pass on your left. From the parking area, you will cross the street to find the kiosk and day use permits for the Rockbound Trail.

Description: There are two different routes available to Umpa Lake, but neither one is maintained or well marked. The one described here is perhaps the more difficult of the two, but the majority of the way is on a marked trail. Only at the end do you mountaineer down to the lake off trail. The only real difficulty here is to look backwards and make mental marks for the return trip. The trail rating is a three due to the mountaineering involved, not to the physical difficulty (more of a 2). If you are not comfortable going off trail, then you should not attempt this hike.

You want to do this hike as soon as the snow has melted and the trails are clear in order to enjoy the fullest of the waterfalls into Umpa Lake. Numerous falls develop from the water flowing above down glaciated rock slabs. In a heavy rain year, the noise from the falls is audible from the launching point from the Tyler Lake Trail. In a lesser rainfall year, the falls are still impressive, and swimming is more comfortable even in July (otherwise you would be wise to wait until August for swimming).

Starting from the trailhead, you have a short ascent before a descent to arrive at Beauty Lake in about 15 minutes. At the lake, follow the signs to the Wilderness Area and walk around the lake to your left, ignoring the sign for the Jeep Trail. Once you leave the lake, follow all posts directing you towards Rockbound Trail. Continue to follow the posts in the direction of Rockbound Pass, reaching the one for Tyler Lake at 2.1 miles. Go right here and follow the Tyler Lake Trail. Shortly after you start on this trail, you will enter into Desolation Wilderness.

Now you start a tough 0.25-mile ascent of 200 feet up a rock gully. Watch carefully for trail markers during the climb. Typically, these markers are piles of small rocks on top of larger rocks. These rock piles, called "ducks," are throughout Desolation Wilderness marking trails across rock surfaces.

At the peak of the gully, look down to your right to see Umpa Lake below. You should be able to both see the lake and hear its waterfalls. Leave Tyler Lake Trail here and make your way down to Umpa Lake. Be sure to turn around during your 200-foot descent to mark distinctive trees or rocks to follow on your return trip. Once at the lake, you will not be able to see your launching point, so you need to have mental marks mid-way down for retracing your steps.

The lake is a great lunch spot, a good fishing possibility, a photographic haven, and a swimming opportunity. You may be surprised to see how many people are also at the lake (unless you go mid-week). Did they all come the way you did? Most likely, they did not. Most locals come via the other route originating from the Twin Lakes Trail. This other route is an easier hike, but more difficult to follow unless you are with someone who has done the hike before. For safety's sake, stick with returning the same way you came.

Hike 27 - Maud Lake
Rockbound Pass Trail
Wrights Lake, CA

Difficulty: 3

Distance: 4.6 miles to lake

Elevation: 640 feet total gain, but more vertical feet with first going up, then down to creek, and then back up again

Directions: From Highway 50 East at Kyburz, continue another 4.8 miles to a left turn onto Wrights Road. Follow this road 8.1 miles into the Wrights Lake Campground. At the Stop sign, continue straight another 0.3 mile to the parking for Rockbound Pass on your left. From the parking area, you cross the street to find the kiosk and day use permits for the Rockbound Trail.

Description: This is a challenging but fun hike with a variety of habitats to explore. Starting from the trailhead, you have a short ascent before a descent to arrive at Beauty Lake in about 15 minutes. At the lake, follow the signs to the Wilderness Area and walk around the lake to your left, ignoring the sign for the Jeep Trail.

Once you leave the lake, follow all posts directing you to Rockbound Trail. Shortly, you will start to enjoy great views of the distant mountain range. Look for the reddish peak and then to its left for the low, saddle area – this is Rockbound Pass. Maud Lake lies below the pass.

Continue to follow the posts in the direction of Rockbound Pass, passing the one for Tyler Lake at 2.1 miles. Shortly after this, you will enter into Desolation Wilderness and a tough ascent of about 0.5

mile. You will arrive at a seasonal pond on your left and then start descending over rock slabs to reach the Jones Fork Silver Creek. This can be a simple "rock hop" crossing, or a very difficult attempt after a heavy rain season. In July of 2006, I had to stop here and turn around, but in June of 2007, I had no problems and was able to continue to Maud Lake.

After crossing the creek, you will ascend over slabs of rocks before reaching Willow Flat. Since it is difficult to follow a trail along rock slabs, conspicuous piles of small rocks have been placed periodically along the way. Look for these rock piles, known as "ducks," to make your way across the slabs.

In Willow Flat, you are welcomed by cooler air, probably a nice breeze, and along with the willows, you have aspens, corn lilies, and ferns. Magnificent rock walls frame the flat, holding in the fresh smell of pines and songs of birds. A small stream nourishes this habitat. You seem to leave it for a climb up and around a large rock, only to return to its shade for a little while longer. When you emerge, a large rock wall ahead confronts you. To your left is a little spur trail, but your trek is up the trail to the top of the rocks.

The 200-foot ascent is difficult, but not too lengthy. Pussypaws and penstemon decorate the rocks. As you near the top, you will pick up the sound of water and can look down to your right to see Silver Creek flowing down a gorge. The trail flattens and you come to the lower part of Maud Lake, which is more like a pond. Continue just a little further to reach the lake itself. If you like to fish, then bring your gear and definitely try your luck.

Less Ambitious Option: Stop at Beauty Lake and enjoy the alpine scenery. This is an easy walk and a nice place to picnic. After a rest, you can continue walking a little further for views of the Crystal Range, and then turn around to return to your car.

Hike 28 - Woods Lake Trail to Winnemucca and Round Top Lakes
Woods Lake Trailhead
Highway 88 Past Caples Lake

Difficulty: 3

Distance: 4.6-mile loop

Elevation: 1135 feet gain from trailhead to Round Top Lake

Directions: Drive East on Highway 88 15.5 miles beyond the intersection with Mormon Emigrant Trail (either take Highway 88 from Jackson, or Highway 50 to Exit 60 in Sly Park to Mormon Emigrant Trail). Find the entrance to Woods Lake Campground on your right just past Caples Lake. Drive 1.0 mile on its asphalt road to the Woods Lake Trailhead Parking area on your right. There is a day use fee for parking ($3.00 in 2007).

Description: Plan on taking this hike in mid- to late-July, depending on the severity of the winter. Give the trail time for the snow to melt and the streams to be more easily crossed, yet still enjoy the wild flowers at their peak.

From the parking area, continue on the asphalt road across the bridge to the trail on your right. Continue 0.1 mile to the marked post for Winnemucca Lake to the left and Round Top Lake to the right. Go in the direction to Winnemucca Lake (the other arm is the return route). Cross the asphalt road and find the trail marker on the opposite side.

The first part of the trail is forested and pleasant with just a slight rise. You will cross a stream and enjoy the shaded, well-maintained trail. Notice the blue diamonds in the trees marking the trail for snowshoeing in the winter. After a mile, you will have gained 325 feet and emerge from your forest shade. Now the views of the distant mountain peaks improve as you hike along the hills of wildflowers, peaking in mid-July. Shortly, you will enter into the Mokelumne Wilderness. To your right, a spur trail takes you down to a small stream. As you continue ahead the last 0.5 mile to Winnemucca Lake, the climb intensifies, gaining another 440 feet, so take your time and enjoy the views.

Winnemucca Lake is a popular destination, also accessible from the Carson Pass Trailhead. It has beautiful blue, clear water and provides a good fishing spot. As you arrive at the lake, you will notice the post marking the trail up to Round Top Lake. After resting at Winnemucca, continue your hike in the direction of Round Top. This section of the hike is just 1.0 mile, and you will climb another 370 feet. Looking back down the trail, you have great views of Winnemucca Lake below and ahead Round Top Peak looms. As you arrive at Round Top Lake, look for the post marking the next leg of your loop in the direction of Woods Lake.

Round Top Lake's water is greener and the lake is smaller than Winnemucca. Still, you will find fish here if you want to try your luck. It will be much cooler at this higher elevation (Round Top Peak is 10,381') and most likely windy. Unless it is a very hot day at the start of your hike, expect to be cold at the lake, so take a jacket along in your pack.

From Round Top Lake, take the 2.0-mile trail down to Woods Lake, also called the Lost Cabin Mine Trail. Starting down, you will enjoy great views ahead. Shortly, you can look down to Caples Lake in the distance. The trail follows numerous streams along its descent. In about a mile, you will arrive at remnants of an old mining camp. Leaving the camp, you will continue downhill, picking up views of Woods Lake below. There is a final stream crossing that could be difficult in a heavy rain year, so be safe crossing it.

Notes: Please be respectful of the rules for Mokelumne Wilderness to leash your dog. By following the rules, you ensure the Forest

Service will continue to allow dogs into the Wilderness Area in the future.

AUGUST

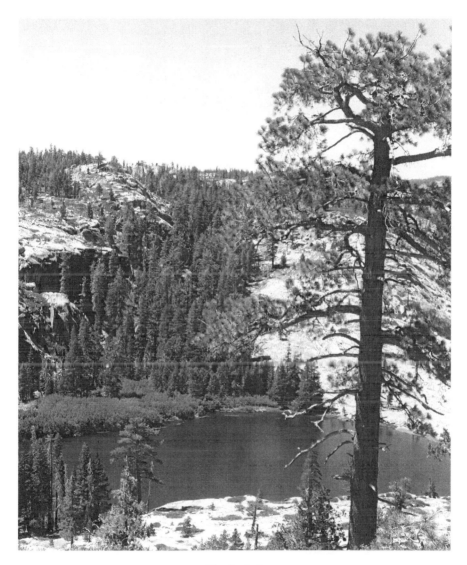

Shealor Lake

AUGUST

In August, you continue with mountain hikes. With luck, you will still enjoy wildflowers in the meadow portion of the hike to Lake Sylvia. As you probably have come to realize, the trails in the mountains are not as easy to follow as the ones in the lower elevations. My son did the Shealor Lake hike and was mostly off-trail, rock scaling down to the lake. You need to carefully spot trail markers on these hikes.

For a good outing this month for those with physical limitations, follow the directions for the hike to Boomerang Lake and do the one-mile Loop Trail at Wrights Lake. This will get you out of the valley heat and into some beautiful surroundings. Additionally, you could consider a revisit to Meeks Creek (Hike 7) for a pleasant hike without the snow.

Hike 29 – Boomerang Lake
Twin Lakes Trail
Wrights Lake Campground

Difficulty: 3
Distance: 3.1 miles to lake
Elevation: 1050 feet gain

Directions: Heading east on Highway 50, continue 4.8 miles past Kyburz to a left turn onto Wrights Road. Travel 8.1 miles to the campground. At the first Stop sign, turn right and go 1.0 mile to the trailhead parking for Twin and Grouse Lakes. If the parking area is full, you will need to return to the Stop sign, turn left, and find the overflow parking area on the left. If you need to park here, then you will add another mile to the hike in both directions. This is a popular trailhead, so get there early for better parking.

Description: You will follow the Twin Lakes Trail to Lower Twin Lake and then continue across its rock dam another 0.5 mile to the more secluded Boomerang Lake. In August, it should be perfect for swimming, so wear your suit under your hiking clothes. While the hike is not terribly long, it involves a lot of climbing, often in areas exposed to the sun, so remember your hat, sunglasses, and sunscreen.

Starting from the parking area, walk through the service gate and down to the trailhead kiosk. Here you can fill out your day permit for entering Desolation Wilderness. You start on the Loop Trail for an easy 0.4 mile before reaching the Twin Lakes Trailhead on your right signed for Twin, Grouse, Island, and Hemlock Lakes.

From here, you start a 140-foot ascent before reaching a saddle. Then you ascend another 300 feet with Grouse Lake's outlet creek on your left. Within a mile, you will reach the wilderness boundary. Shortly thereafter, you come to a trail post indicating Grouse Lake to the right and Twin Lake to the left. Follow in the direction of Twin Lake.

Soon you will cross the Grouse Lake creek, and depending on the previous rainy season, the crossing is either a simple rock hop or a more difficult challenge. After making the crossing, turn around and make mental notes on where you came across and where the trail is on the other side for your return trip. It is easy to run into difficulties on your return if you do not cross at the same place.

After the creek crossing, you start ascending again over rock slabs. Here you need to look ahead for the next rock piles marking the trail to find your way. These piles of small rocks are "ducks", and they mark many of the trails in Desolation. Over the 1.7 miles from the trail post to Lower Twin Lake, you will be climbing steadily. When you reach the Twin Lake outlet creek, you will hear its waterfall and see it on your left. At this point, you need to carefully find the trail, which is not the spur taking you over to the creek. Instead, the actual trail bends away from the creek and then ascends more over rocks before bending back towards the creek. Always look ahead for the trail markers made from rock piles. If at any point you are not certain of the trail, then backtrack to the last known marker, and look ahead more diligently for the next marker. Do not advance without being certain of your path. It is a popular trail, so you can always wait for people coming down to see their path, or for someone else coming up the trail so you can follow.

After this last climb, you come to a welcome descent to a little pond. From here, you cross the creek on rock steps and follow the trail up to Lower Twin Lake. When you reach the lake, turn around and make notes as to where the trail ends at the lake. Identify a certain tree or large rock to be your reminder for your return.

Lower Twin is the most popular lake along this trail. If it is not busy, then enjoy a moment to relax here and fish. Otherwise, you may want to continue on to the less popular Boomerang Lake, a short 0.4

mile away. To reach Boomerang, cross Twin Lake's rock dam to pick up the trail again. The dam is on your left as you face Twin Lake. (In an extremely heavy rainfall year, the dam may be difficult to cross. If water is flowing over it, then try finding a safer crossing downstream and then come back up from the other side to find the trail again.)

The trail takes you along Twin Lake's western shore and then reaches a rock gully to climb. In a short amount of time, you will reach the petite Boomerang Lake. Here you can enjoy a pleasant swim and lunch. If it is too crowded, you can opt for Upper Twin Lake directly opposite Boomerang, a short distance from the trail you came from. There is no actual trail down to Upper Twin, but it is easy to make your way down to it to enjoy its seclusion.

More Ambitious Option: Continue a short 0.2 miles beyond Boomerang Lake, and you will find Island Lake. This is a popular lake for fly-fishing.

Less Ambitious Option: Instead of taking the Twin Lake trail, continue on the Loop Trail around the Wrights Lake Recreation Area. This is a peaceful 1.0 mile walk, crossing a bridge from where you can look down to see fish below. Visitors like to kayak or canoe through the waterways that line the trail.

Hike 30 – Lake Sylvia
Lyons Creek Trailhead
Wrights Road

Difficulty: 3

Distance: 5.0 miles to lake (my pedometer and topographic map say 4.6 miles, but the trailhead map says 5.0 miles)

Elevation: 1340 feet gain from trailhead to lake

Directions: From Highway 50 heading east, 4.8 miles past Kyburz, turn left onto Wrights Road. Go 4.0 miles to the Lyons Creek Trailhead parking area on your right. There is plenty of parking here, but it is very popular, so if the lot is full you can continue just a little further and find more parking at the creek. At the trailhead, you will find a kiosk with a map and day passes; you need to fill out a pass to enter the wilderness area.

Description: This hike parallels Lyons Creek as you ascend to the lake. The creek, always within earshot, has several access spots for breaks, with sections of falls over larger granite slabs. The first part of the hike goes through meadows of corn lilies and lupine, with other wildflowers mixed in, filling a color palette. While the meadows are beautiful, unfortunately everything that can bite seems to be successful doing so throughout your journey – carry and use your bug spray generously.

After 1.9 miles, you will reach a marker post indicating Bloodsucker Lake (named for its leech inhabitants) to the left. Your destination, Lake Sylvia, is straight ahead. However, a brief 0.1-mile side trip in the direction of Bloodsucker, takes you to a nice spot along the creek for a break before returning to the main trail. At 3.0 miles, you enter Desolation Wilderness and most of the climbing ensues.

At 4.0 miles, you will cross Lyons Creek (if there is too much water, look upstream a short way for an easier crossing). At 4.6 miles, you will come to the marker post for Lyons Lake to the left. Lake Sylvia is straight from here another 0.4 mile. You will cross the Lyons Lake outlet creek and then the outlet from an unnamed lake before reaching Lake Sylvia. All of the creek crossings should be simple rock hops, depending on the previous winter's rain and snowfall. In August, you can swim in Lake Sylvia. Fishing is good here also. For prime viewing of wildflowers, July or early August is best. Take time to walk around the lake for different views. From Lake Sylvia, it is popular to climb up to 9983' Pyramid Peak, so with luck you can sit at lakeside and watch someone else make the effort.

Consider a return trip here in a couple of months to enjoy some beautiful fall colors. Later in the year, it can get cold at the lake, so bring extra layers for fall hikes.

Hike 31 - Dardanelles Lake
Big Meadow Trailhead
Tahoe Rim Trail

Difficulty: 3
Distance: 3.5 miles to lake
Elevation: Three climbs in to lake of 250, 535, and
100 feet, and 180-foot climb out

Directions: Head east on Highway 50 towards Lake Tahoe and then after making the summit, continue another 4.0 miles down to the junction with Highway 89. Turn right onto Highway 89 and go 5.25 miles to the Big Meadow Trailhead parking area on the left. The trail starts at the bottom of the parking area, heading back across Highway 89.

Description: This is a popular trail, but do not let all the cars deter you. A number of trail users are joggers out for a morning run, so they will be finishing early and leaving the trail open for hikers and mountain bikers. From the parking area, find the trail at the lower end and walk 0.1 mile back to the highway. Carefully cross the highway to find the trailhead for the Big Meadow portion of the Tahoe Rim Trail.

The first part of the trail climbs 250 feet for 0.4 mile. You will find a fork in the trail at the crest of the hill. The left fork takes you to Scotts Lake. Stay to the right here for Dardanelles Lake and continue into aptly named Big Meadow. The meadow crossing is about 0.2 mile and a pleasant relief after the initial climb.

After enjoying the meadow, the trail starts ascending again through the forest cover. The climb of 535 feet covers a distance of 1.2 miles and it can be dry and dusty in August. You will be relieved to reach the crest of the hill and ready to start a short descent of 0.2 mile to a trail marker post. If you stay straight, you will continue on to Round Lake. For Dardanelles Lake, take the trail on the right signed Christmas Valley.

Hike 0.2 mile on this leg and find the trail going left across a stream. It may not be marked, so look carefully for the path to the left. Now enjoy the last 1.2 miles of this hike, crossing two more streams and paralleling another for a while. Along the way, cross through a small meadow, site a large Juniper tree along the trail, and absorb the great views. Only at the end, there is a short 100-foot climb to the lake.

The lake has clear, cool water, probably too cool for a swim, but you can enjoy a little foot soaking or try some fishing for lake trout. A granite cliff lines Dardanelles' south bank. Walk around to the north side and picnic along the flatter granite slabs. Your return hike will be easier with only the 0.2-mile ascent of 180 feet to confront.

For your return drive, you may want to consider continuing on Highway 89 south to its intersection with Highway 88 in less than 6 miles. Turn right here towards Jackson. This route, although 15 miles longer, will allow you to avoid the busy Lake Tahoe return traffic on Highway 50 and the inevitable backups in Placerville. It also affords a great view into the Kirkwood valley, down to Red Lake and the Carson Pass.

Hike 32 - Shealor Lake
Highway 88 near Silver Lake

Difficulty: 2

Distance: 1 mile to lake

Elevation: 238 feet climb from trailhead into lake;
  470 feet climb out from lake

Before the hike: Stop at **Naughty Pines Kitchen** in Pollock Pines for a nice breakfast. The restaurant has an outdoor area for dining with your dog. At Exit 60 turn left under freeway and then left onto Pony Express Trail to 6404 (on your left). (530) 644-2300

Directions: From Highway 50 in Pollock Pines, take Exit 60 for Sly Park Road. When you exit the freeway, take a right onto Sly Park Road and continue 4.6 miles. Make a left onto Mormon Emigrant Trail and go about 25 miles to its end at Highway 88. Make a left and head east on 88 for 6 miles and locate the Shealor Lake Trailhead parking on your left.

Description: Although this is a short hike, the hike in is slow, taking about 45 minutes. The trail starts with a climb of 238 feet on a well-marked path. At the top of the climb, you can enjoy the great views before starting the 470-foot drop to the lake on a very rocky path. Take your time on the descent to be sure of your footing on the loose rocks. Also, look carefully for the trail markings, such as the rock piled "ducks" and other hiker's footprints.

This is a very pretty hike with views of your destination lake early in your descent. Seeing the lake early on fooled our son, Jake, on his first attempt at this hike, and he just started down towards it, leaving the trail and making for a difficult descent down rocks. So do not let its sighting lure you off-trail. Stay focused and you will safely make it down. When you arrive at the bottom, make a mental note of where the trail emerges for your return trip.

The lake itself has nice clear water for swimming. You can walk around to its eastern shore and see numerous campsites for backpackers. You can also venture from the lake and find a pond beyond it (visible on your hike in to the lake).

The return 470-foot climb is not as difficult as you would think, as there are many switchbacks making for an easy ascent. With the higher elevations and cooler temperatures in the Kirkwood area, this is a good destination on a hot summer afternoon to escape the valley.

SEPTEMBER

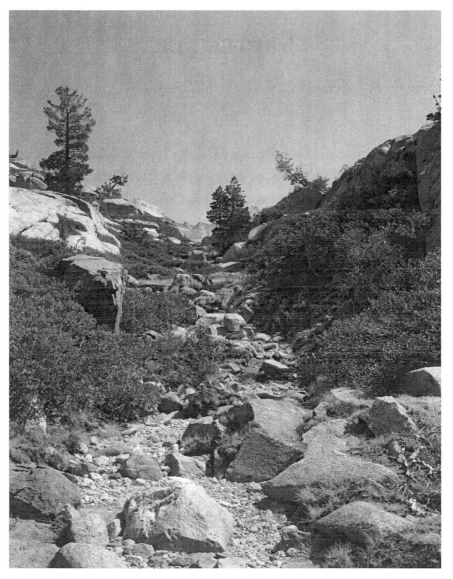

First gully on climb to Gertrude Lake

SEPTEMBER

This month you will have the first difficulty level '4' hike with the one to Gertrude Lake and its many gully ascents. The climb up to Lover's Leap is steep, but not very long. With the hike to Pearl Lake, you will share a part of the trail with 4-wheel drive vehicles on the Barrett Jeep Trail. It is fun to watch them maneuver their vehicles over the rocky, narrow trail.

For an easy hike, choose Gerle Creek, which not only is good for those with physical limitations, but also fun for children with its interpretive signs explaining how the Indians used nature's bounty for their food, shelter, clothing, and medicines.

You may also want to consider a return trip to University Falls (Hike 11) after Labor Day Weekend and watch the locals go down the waterslides. Maybe you will be tempted to try the slides yourself.

Hike 33 - Lover's Leap
Camp Sacramento

Difficulty: 2

Distance: 1.4 miles from parking area to Lover's Leap

Elevation: 500-foot ascent (steepest last 0.4 mile)

Directions: From Strawberry on Highway 50, continue another 3.0 miles east to Camp Sacramento on your right. Turn into the camp on the dirt road and just past the bridge find the Lover's Leap Trail parking on your left. There is space for about six vehicles here. Do not park in the campground or on the right side's area after the bridge, since this is a reserved area for campers at the resort. If the parking area is full, you can return to Highway 50 and find a large turnout you can use and then walk into the camp.

Description: Your first view of Lover's Leap will be in Strawberry. Look up to the right to see its sheer face. The hike from here would be imposing, but by driving another 3.0 miles up the highway, the hike from Camp Sacramento is less of a trek.

From the parking area, walk up the dirt road into the camp. Walk past the camp store, heading in the direction of Strawberry. Just beyond Cabin 52, you will find the Lover's Leap trailhead (0.15 mile from the parking area). The first part of the walk is through a shaded riparian forest of alders, aspen, and pines, along with native brush and a wide selection of wildflowers. Within 0.25 mile, you will arrive at a series of streams. There are also two side trails marked with XP posts, designating cross-country trails. The first of these points is to your left and the second one is to the right. In both cases, continue straight to remain on the Lover's Leap trail. A few minutes beyond the streams, stop and look out across the canyon for a great view of Horsetail Falls.

After a mile of leisurely strolling, you will have easily gained 250 feet. You will gain the remaining 250 feet in the next 0.4 mile. This portion of the trail leaves the shade and you will start climbing over rocks, switch backing your way up the grade. At points, the trail becomes confusing with faint spurs to distract you. You need to look ahead to find the more well traveled path and stick to it. When you feel a need to stop for a rest, take in the spectacular views. You are almost to the top now, with the remaining part less strenuous. When you arrive, you will see a sign on a tree to mark Lover's Leap. In addition, the sign reminds you **DO NOT THROW ROCKS** over the side, since rock climbers frequent the area and rocks could kill them.

While the hike up to the summit may have been a heart throbber, the rewarding views are well worth the effort. Take time to look around at the 360-degree sites, including 9983' Pyramid Peak and 9235' Ralston Peak. Look down to Highway 50 and Strawberry. Do not go too close to the edge and do not allow children to run around, with an obvious danger to an accidental fall. When you are ready to leave, be sure to return on the trail that you arrived on. Another trail down is also available, but this one will take you down to Strawberry and it would be a long walk back to your car. To be safe, make a note of your return route as soon as you arrive.

Hike 34 - Pearl Lake
Barrett Lake Trail
Wrights Lake Recreation Area

Difficulty: 3

Distance: 4.7 miles to lake

Elevation: About 500 feet variation in heights although
"ups and downs" make it seem more extreme

Directions: Heading East on Highway 50, you continue 4.8 miles beyond Kyburz and make a left turn onto Wrights Road. Follow Wrights Road 8.1 miles into the campground. At the Stop sign, continue another 0.3 mile to the Rockbound Pass trailhead parking area on the left. The actual trailhead is across the road. You do not need a day permit for hiking to Pearl Lake, as it is not in Desolation Wilderness.

Description: The best part of this hike is sharing the Jeep portion of the journey with Off Highway Vehicles (OHVs) and watching them maneuver over the rocks and tree roots. The trail is open for OHVs once the ground is dry, while day hikers can go in earlier. If you do not want to share with OHVs then plan on doing this hike earlier in the season when it is only open to hikers.

From the trailhead kiosk, you start on the Rockbound Pass trail and hike 0.5 mile to Beauty Lake. From the lake, you will see a trail marker indicating the Jeep Trail to your left. You walk about 800 feet on this trail before intersecting with the Barrett Lake Trail. Head to your right on the jeep trail, making a note for your return trip of this side trail back to Beauty Lake (if you miss it on your return, you will just continue on the road trail to Dark Lake and then to the parking area for Rockbound Pass).

Once on the jeep trail, you will see immediately a small pond on your left. You will follow the jeep trail slowly downhill until reaching a creek crossing for Jones Fork Silver Creek. By September, this crossing should be easy enough, but if there is still too much water, look upstream at some large boulders to help you safely across.

After crossing the creek, you will start an ascent with the creek following down below the trail on your right. The trail eventually leaves the creek and continues ascending. When you finally reach the top, you reach a flat area called Mortimer Flat. From this flat, look along the main trail to your left for a side trail that takes us to Pearl Lake. (The last time I hiked this, the side trail was marked with three blue ribbons on trees.) From the trailhead to this side trail, you will have gone about 2.6 miles.

Leaving the Jeep Trail behind, this next part of the trail is quiet and very pretty, with pines to shade and meadows of wildflowers. You will enjoy a little downhill meandering before starting another ascent. When you reach the top of this hill, you can look down to a private lake below. The trail then starts downhill, arriving at the fence line for the private land.

Shortly after reaching the fence line, there is a spur trail on your right marked with rock piles. This spur will take you to the main trail to Pearl Lake. If you miss the spur, just continue along the fence line and arrive at the private house. Here you will easily see the Pearl Lake sign pointing you to the main trail for the 0.5-mile hike into the lake.

Pearl Lake does not get many hikers, so it is a peaceful lunch spot. Do not forget to bring your camera so you can photograph this pretty, alpine lake with its lilies, rock dam, and awesome reflections from the surrounding trees. On your trek back, you can take time to enjoy the distant peaks of the Crystal Range.

Share with: OHVs

Hike 35 - Gertrude Lake
Rockbound Pass Trail
Wrights Lake Recreation Area

Difficulty: 4

Distance: 4.2 miles to lake

Elevation: 1040 feet gain to lake

Directions: From Highway 50 East at Kyburz, continue another 4.8 miles to a left turn onto Wrights Road. Follow this road 8.1 miles into the Wrights Lake Campground. At the Stop sign, continue straight another 0.3 mile to the parking for Rockbound Pass on your left. From the parking area, you cross the road to find the kiosk and day-use permits for the Rockbound Trail.

Description: For the first 2.0 miles, the climb is a moderate 300 feet making for a good warm-up for the second half of the hike. Follow all signs for Rockbound Pass until you reach the post pointing to Tyler Lake to your right (about one hour of hiking). Turn here to leave the Rockbound Pass Trail and start on Tyler Lake Trail. The trail briefly passes through a flat with alders before starting its climb to the Desolation Wilderness boundary.

Avoid all spurs taking you to the right, instead heading straight until you reach the boundary sign. At the sign look for the trail on your right and start your ascent. This is the first of three gullies to climb on this hike. Avoid spurs to the right and look ahead for rock piles known as "ducks" to guide your way. This first gully is about a 200-foot ascent. At the top, you can look down to your right to Umpa Lake and Wrights Lake in the distance.

From here, the trail heads briefly down hill to your left. Then you start the 140-foot climb up the second gully. At the top, you have a pleasant, but short, walk through a forested saddle before arriving at the final gully. This third gully is a 75-foot ascent and again tops out at a flat, forested area. You then reach another rocky climb of about 235 feet over rocky slabs; the trail is faint in spots before you reach a pond on your left (could be dry by now).

The pond area is pleasant, forested with hemlocks, the trail following the natural runoffs from spring. By this time of year, the trail will be dry and easier to follow. Enjoy this section for its short span and then prepare for another rocky climb. The trail can be difficult to follow, so make sure you clearly see your path or the next "ducks" marking your way before proceeding forward. Soon now, you will arrive at shallow Gertrude Lake.

When you start your return trip, after about 0.25 mile, look on your right for a field of willow bushes and a spur trail taking you to Tyler's grave with its white marble headstone. Tyler was a ranch hand who died in a snowstorm in 1882 and honored with a final resting spot in this beautiful setting.

Enjoy the rest of the hike back to your car, now mostly downhill. Great viewing spots abound on your trip out. The wildflowers are long gone now, replaced with the beginnings of autumn brown and gold grasses. In another month, more fall colors will be on display.

Less Ambitious Option: You can start the hike as described and in approximately 45 minutes (1.6 miles), you will reach a post directing you to Rockbound Pass to the left and Wrights Lake to the right. Take the direction to Wrights Lake on a nice little trail down to the recreation area. From here, you can take the trail along the eastern shoreline, and return to the main road. Walk the 0.3 mile down the road back to your car for a total hike of approximately three miles.

Hike 36 - Gerle Creek
Crystal Basin Recreation Area
Ice House Road

Difficulty: 1

Distance: 0.5-0.7 mile one-way

Elevation: This is a flat trail, with only a 10-foot elevation change

Directions: From Highway 50 going east, turn left onto Ice House Road immediately after crossing the bridge over the South Fork American River (about 22 miles east of Placerville). Follow Ice House Road 26.5 miles to a left turn into Gerle Creek (this will be 2.8 miles beyond the right turn for Loon Lake). Drive 1.0 mile into the campground and through the campsites to reach the day use parking area (no fee for the day use area).

Description: Gerle Creek offers one of the best interpretive trails in this area. Take the time to read all of the markers, as they are full of interesting information.

From the parking area, locate the sign for the Lake Shore Trail. This trail goes 0.7 mile to the dam. For most of the distance (0.5 mile), the Lake Shore Trail joins with the Summer Harvest Trail. The Summer Harvest Trail is an interpretive trail with 14 markers describing each scene and the ways the Indians used nature for making their food, medicines, homes, clothes, and trade items. The markers give you complete descriptions of the scenes, and suggest points for you to smell a tree, or touch a grinding rock. The trail is wheelchair accessible, flat, and shaded. Benches are available along the shoreline.

The Summer Harvest Trail ends at the last post comparing life then and now. You can continue the final way to the dam on a lesser path (not suitable for disabled travelers).

The dam works to form a peaceful lake out of Gerle Creek. Enjoy your stay at the reservoir, picnic, or fish for brown trout. Motorboats are not allowed on this lake, making for an idyllic site for canoeing.

OCTOBER

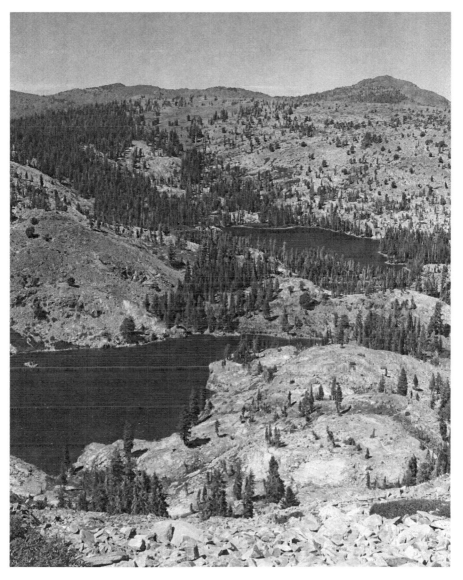

View down to Ralston, Tamarack, and Cagwin Lakes

OCTOBER

This month you can tackle a difficulty '5' hike with a climb to the top of Mt. Tallac. Only the most physically fit should attempt this strenuous outing. An easier venture into Desolation is the hike to Tamarack, Ralston, and Cagwin Lakes. The pretty hike to Lake Margaret offers a variety of scenery. Start your day early for the drive is a little farther and the crowds arrive in the afternoon. For those with physical limitations, you have the Nevada Beach trip. October offers something for everyone.

You may also consider a return trip to Caples Creek (Hike 23) to enjoy the fall colors. Finally, if you return to Camp Richardson and the Taylor Creek Visitor Center (Hike 22) you may be fortunate to time the spawning of the Kokanee salmon and rainbow trout.

Hike 37 - Tamarack, Ralston, and Cagwin Lakes
Echo Lakes Trail

Difficulty: 2
Distance: 4.1 miles to lakes
Elevation: 380 feet gain

Directions: Heading East on Highway 50, continue 6.0 miles beyond Twin Bridges, making a left onto Johnson Pass Road. Drive 0.5 mile to a left onto Echo Lakes Road. Continue 1.0 mile down Echo Lakes to the large parking area above the resort. There is both a paved and a dirt parking area. A trail down to the resort starts from the dirt parking lot, signed on a tree. You walk steeply down the trail (100-foot descent in 0.15 mile) to reach the resort.

Description: Starting at the resort, walk across the dam to a kiosk with day use permits. From here, climb a short distance to a plateau with a trail coming in on the right. Your Echo Lakes Trail heads to the left here to parallel Lower and Upper Echo Lakes for 2.5 miles. This part of the hike is relatively flat, with little rolling hills and one switchback. While you hike, you can look down on the summer lake homes with envy. When you leave the lakes behind, you continue another 0.6 mile to reach the boundary for Desolation Wilderness. From here, continue another 0.5 mile to a post on your left signed for Tamarack Lake.

The trail down to Tamarack is a short 0.25 mile and a little vague at times. When you reach the lake, be sure to note trail signs for your return trip. Tamarack is the largest of the three lakes in the Ralston Peak basin, also the most popular to visit. To leave the crowds, continue on the trail along the lake's eastern shore. In a short distance, it moves away from the lake and then climbs up to your left over some rocks. When you reach the top, you can look down to see Ralston Lake below. Ralston is 0.2 mile from Tamarack Lake.

At Ralston, you can cross its rock dam to reach its eastern shore with nice sandy beach areas. The water is deep and perfect for swimming or fishing. On the western shore, there are large boulders at the water's edge. Ralston is a very pretty lake with a view up to Ralston Peak at its southern end.

After your stay at Ralston, continue a short 0.1 mile to Cagwin Lake. To reach Cagwin, you head away from Ralston from its dam end to find the trail. In a short distance, you will see Cagwin Lake down to your right. Cagwin is the smallest of the three lakes, but more secluded with fewer visitors. Not as deep as Ralston, there is more vegetation in the water. From Cagwin Lake, return to Ralston and then to Tamarack for your trip home.

Less Ambitious Option: Plan to do this hike before Labor Day and take the water taxi at the Echo Lakes Resort. This cuts out the first 2.5 miles of the hike. The taxi costs $10.00/person and $4.00/dog one-way (2007 prices). Call ahead for times (530) 659-7207. The taxi does not run after Labor Day Weekend.

Hike 38 - Lake Margaret
Kirkwood, CA

Difficulty: 2
Distance: 5 miles roundtrip
Elevation: 200 feet gain

Directions: From Highway 50 in Pollock Pines, take Exit 60 for Sly Park Road As you exit the freeway, you will take a right onto Sly Park Road and continue 4.6 miles. Here make a left onto Mormon Emigrant Trail and go about 25 miles to its end at Highway 88. Make a left and head east on 88 to Kirkwood.

Continue past the ski resort on your right and the Kirkwood Cross Country and Snowshoe Center on your left. The next left (0.1 mile from the Cross Country center) is the entrance to the parking area for Lake Margaret. There is ample parking here, but it can get crowded in the afternoons.

Description: The hike into Lake Margaret is just 2.5 miles, making it one of the easiest hikes to an alpine lake in the Sierra. This is a scenic hike through various habitats, with streams, marshes, aspen groves, and granite rocks to traverse. There are log crossings at various points, but if you wear hiking sandals, you can easily wade through the water to avoid the logs.

The trail is well marked with signs, blazes on trees (blazes are obvious scars on the tree's trunk due to removal of a strip of the bark, slightly above eye level), and rock piles ("ducks") marking the way over rocky areas where the trail disappears. There are numerous spur trails to fool you at times, but if you look ahead for the next marker, you can easily stay on the wider main trail.

Starting from the parking area you will see the trailhead sign and start a nice 100-foot descent. Quickly the sounds of running water and singing birds replace the noise from the highway. You will reach water quickly and can look over a cliff at a stream below. At 0.5 mile, you will see a spur trail on your left taking you to a peaceful stream and meadow area. The main trail goes to the right here.

At 0.75 mile, the trail borders a large rock wall. The main trail goes to the left here away from the wall. There is a signpost to indicate the trail, but it was broken the last time I visited. Shortly you will come to one of the log crossings with an extremely wide log for your use. From here, the trail starts uphill and then around a large rock formation. The trail goes to the left around the rocky area and arrives at a small pond (may be dry).

From the pond, the trail goes to the right, keeping the pond on your left. You will find blazes on trees, and "ducks" to mark your way. At 1.5 miles, you will arrive at a larger pond. Continue now across rocks and through a grove of large aspens to the final water crossing. After making the crossing, look for the trail to your right taking you uphill. You have a short ascent over rocks to arrive at the plateau and then an easy walk into the lake. It takes about 1.5 hours to reach the lake. Relax and enjoy the lake before your return trip, remembering you have that 100-foot ascent at the end back to your car. On your trip out, look for a great view of 10,381' Round Top Peak in the distance.

This is a great hike for your dog, with lots of water and open space to enjoy. Try to start early in the morning to avoid the afternoon crowds. In a year with low rainfall, and no late snow, you can come here in mid-June and enjoy the greenery and fresh wildflowers.

Hike 39 - Nevada Beach
Zephyr Cove, NV

Difficulty: 1
Distance: 1-2 miles
Elevation: Flat

Directions: From Stateline, continue into Nevada on Highway 50 past the casinos towards Carson City for 1.6 miles. Turn Left at Elks Point Road in Zephyr Cove. Go 0.5 mile and park along the shoulder at the park entrance.

Description: Start walking along the bike trail in either direction. There are trails throughout the park. You can walk towards the lake and enjoy Nevada Beach, with nice views across the water. From there, you can head into the meadows along the trails, reading some informational signs about the Indians once inhabiting the area. The trails are all flat, making for a leisurely stroll.

This is a fun place to visit in the winter also when the snow has blanketed the meadow. You can still generally walk the trails easily enough without snowshoes since the terrain is so flat. This is a year round fun family excursion.

Hike 40 - Mt. Tallac via Floating Island Lake Camp Richardson, CA

Difficulty: 5

Distance: 1.7 miles to Floating Island Lake

2.5 miles to Cathedral Lake

4.7 miles to Mt. Tallac

Elevation: 3300 feet elevation gain

Directions: In South Lake Tahoe, at the junction of Highways 50 and 89, continue straight on Highway 89. Continue 3.9 miles and make a left turn in the direction of Mt. Tallac Trailhead (at 3.2 miles you will see the Lake Tahoe Visitor Center on the right where you can pick up a Wilderness Day Permit; however, usually these are also available at the trailhead).

Follow the signs pointing to Mt. Tallac, first a left at 0.4 mile and then a right at a second fork. From here, drive 0.4 mile to the trailhead parking area. This is a popular summer hike and the parking can be full in peak season, but in late October, there should plenty of spaces.

Description: This is an uphill hike with a lot of elevation gain. In addition, the footing is difficult with many loose rocks to ascend. You should plan on more time than normal to make the 4.7 miles to the peak of Mt. Tallac. My normal mountain hiking time is 2.0 miles per hour, but on this hike, on the steeper parts my time was closer to 1.0 mile per hour. Be sure to bring along a good camera and a map of Desolation Wilderness and seriously consider hiking poles for balance.

From the parking area, you will start your ascent with a sweat-breaking 250-foot rocky climb before slightly leveling. After another 100 feet of climbing, you will emerge with a great view of Fallen Leaf Lake and Lake Tahoe. After 0.5 mile, the trail leaves the ridge and you head away from Fallen Leaf Lake and another ridge. Leaving that ridge, the hike is less rocky and you pass a stream. At 1.7 miles, you will reach the Wilderness border and Floating Island Lake just beyond. Occasionally, mats of grass break away from the lake's shore, forming floating island mats, giving the lake its name.

Leaving Floating Island, continue on the trail 0.8 mile to Cathedral Lake. Just before reaching the lake, there will be a post marking a trail down to Fallen Leaf Lake. Continue on to the smaller Cathedral Lake, named appropriately for the cathedral-like rock mass above its western shore, known as Cathedral Peak. Take a nice rest here, because soon you will start the steepest part of the climb. You are now over half way to Mt. Tallac, but have only gained a third of the elevation at this point so the climb ahead will be much steeper.

You leave Cathedral Lake in the direction of Cathedral Peak. Climbing above the lake, you have great views back down to Cathedral and Fallen Leaf Lakes. The climb here is difficult, but it will shortly worsen. Look for rock "ducks" marking the trail, ascending to a point where you can see the path ahead climbing steeply up the rocky face of Mt. Tallac's southeast ridge. This part of the trail is extremely steep, almost vertical at times, and very slippery with small rocks. Take your time making your way up. If your calves start to hurt, then concentrate on planting your foot with the heel rather than the toes. This should help to stretch the calves.

When you finally reach the top of this section, you will hike out a short distance to a trail. You will go right here, but make a note that there is also a trail going to your left. On your return trip, be sure to remember this spot so you do not continue hiking down the slope. You will need to make a left turn on your return to attain the correct trail, so look back now and remember this area and make a mental note of the return route.

You have now completed the steepest portion of the hike, gaining another 1000 feet, but ascents remain, eventually gaining another 1000 feet. Your reward is the great views to the west of distant peaks of the Crystal Range and lakes lying below them. Towards the end of the climb, you will reach a junction with the trail leading down to Gilmore Lake. Turn right here for the final 0.2 mile and 200 feet vertical gain to reach the peak of Mt. Tallac.

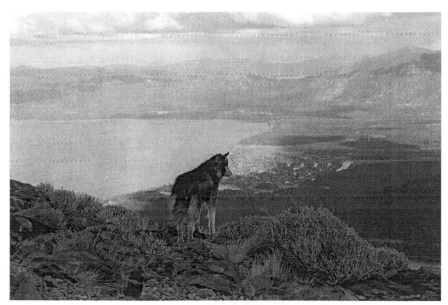

Toots looking out from the top of Mt. Tallac

From this point, the views are great both to the east with Lake Tahoe in site, and to the west down to Gilmore Lake, Susie Lake, and

Lake Aloha. Hopefully, you have packed in a good map of Desolation Wilderness to help you to identify the distant peaks, mountain ranges, and lakes. While the trek was strenuous, the rewarding views make it all worthwhile.

Note that you are at 9735' at the peak of Mt. Tallac and the weather can be changeable. You will want warm clothing with you and rain gear. Do not attempt this hike if thunderstorms are in the forecast. It will be very windy at the peak. Also, remember to take time on the hike back down because the steep sections will be extremely slippery. If you start to fall, try to land on your rear to avoid injuring a wrist or a knee. Take all precautions to make this a safe journey.

NOVEMBER

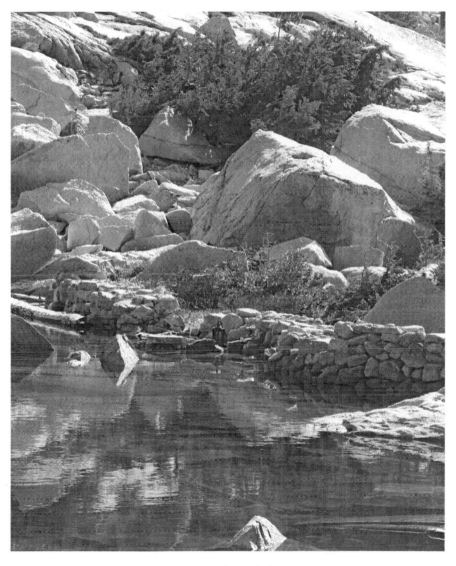

Dam at Smith Lake

November

This month you have the last hike to the high country and into Desolation Wilderness. Unless there is early snow, the hike to Grouse, Hemlock, and Smith Lakes should be perfect in this month's cooler weather. You have a forty-foot waterfall to visit on the Codfish Creek Falls hike. Although this is a difficulty '1' hike, I do not recommend it for those with physical disabilities since there are narrow parts to the trail with steep drop offs. However, it should be a fun hike for children. For the easiest hike, try the trail at Jenkinson Lake in Sly Park. Finally, in Placerville, you discover the unpaved portion of their bike trail, known as the El Dorado Trail.

Hike 41 - Grouse, Hemlock, and Smith Lakes
Wrights Lake Recreation Area

Difficulty: 4

Distance: 2.1 miles to Grouse

             2.6 miles to Hemlock

             3.1 miles to Smith

Elevation: 1740 feet gain from trailhead to Smith Lake

Directions: On Highway 50 in Fresh Pond, make the left turn to Mill Run Ranger Station to pick of a day use permit for Desolation Wilderness (they will not be available at the trailhead in November). Back on Highway 50, heading east, you will continue to Kyburz and then 4.8 miles beyond to the left turn onto Wrights Road.

Go 8.1 miles on Wrights Road into the Wrights Lake Recreation Area. Turn right at the Stop sign and go 1.0 mile down the narrow road to the Twin Lakes Trailhead Parking Area. This is the off-season, so there will be plenty of parking.

Description: I like doing this more difficult hike in November, with the cooler weather making it more pleasurable. If snow threatens, then postpone doing this trip.

Starting from the parking area, walk down the road and past the service gate to find the Loop Trail starting on your right and the Twin Lakes information board. Follow the Loop Trail 0.4 mile to the signed trail for Twin, Grouse, Island, and Hemlock Lakes going to the right.

From here, you start a 140-foot ascent before reaching a saddle. Then you ascend another 150 feet to emerge at a trail of rock slabs, often difficult to follow. Keep the Grouse Lake's outlet creek on your left, climbing another 170 feet. Within 1.0 mile and another 100 feet, you will reach the wilderness boundary. Shortly thereafter, you come to a trail post indicating Grouse Lake to the right and Twin Lake to the left. Follow in the direction of Grouse Lake.

The trail starts over rock slabs, forcing you to look ahead for rock "ducks" marking your way. The trail then veers right as you ascend a gully. The trail flattens for a while, then climbs steeply, ending at the Grouse Lake outlet creek. You need to cross the creek to find the trail on the other side and then continue your climb. You will have gained another 630 feet to reach Grouse Lake. Grouse is a pretty lake, good for swimming in August and fishing in November.

The trail continues along Grouse's northern shore, and then shortly past the lake, it veers left, uphill another 240 feet, in a northeast direction, reaching smaller Hemlock Lake in 0.5 mile. From Hemlock, the trail follows its western shore in a southeastern direction another 0.5 mile and another 310 feet to Smith Lake. The trail in to Smith Lake is difficult to follow in sections so you must choose your trail carefully.

Smith Lake sports clear water, good fishing, and great views down to Wrights Lake, and even to Union Valley Reservoir in the distant Crystal Basin Recreation Area. Enjoy the journey downhill on your return.

Hike 42 (A) - Jenkinson Lake Shoreline Trail
Sly Park, CA

Difficulty: 1

Distance: 8.5-mile loop hike around the lake or you can just do a portion (i.e., 2 miles to Pine Cone Campground and a visit to Miwok Trail, makes about 4.5 miles in and out)

Elevation: Flat trail around lake, with only about 100-foot change in elevation overall

Directions: Heading East on Highway 50, take the second Pollock Pines exit (Exit 60) for Sly Park Road. At the end of the off-ramp, turn right onto Sly Park Road and travel 4.6 miles to Mormon Emigrant Trail, and make a left. Go 0.2 mile to the trailhead and parking area on your left. If the parking is full, continue further on the road and more areas are available.

Description: If you are starting to feel the stresses of the upcoming holiday season, give yourself a time out and enjoy a relaxing walk amongst the pines at Jenkinson Lake. Please note that dogs cannot swim in the lake as the water is for domestic use.

From the Shoreline Trail trailhead, start in a clockwise direction around the lake towards the marina. You will pass the marina, launching area, and day-use picnic area along the way.

At times, the trail is confusing with many spurs taking you up to restrooms or down to picnic tables. Remember, it is a shoreline trail, so when in doubt, stick to the trail closest to the lake. When you reach the other end of the lake, there is sign pointing to Pine Cone Campground to the right or straight to the Miwok Trail. To stay with the shoreline trail, go in the direction of Pine Cone Campground. The trail takes you along the shore in front of the campground.

The side trip to the Miwok Trail is well worth it. This is a self-guided nature trail with many markers along the path labeling the trees, plants, and exhibits. A map at the entrance shows the two main loops making up the trail, but in addition, there is another Logger's Loop you will find along the way. All of these trails are easy and worth doing.

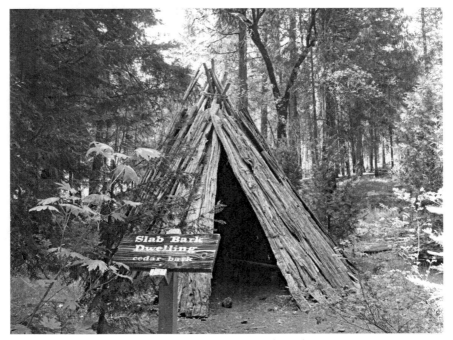

Bark Dwelling at Miwok Trail

After the hike: Consider a side trip to **Sierra Vista Winery**. They have a number of outdoor tables and a great panoramic view. From Mormon Emigrant Trail, return to Sly Park Road, but then turn left towards Pleasant Valley. Continue 7.1 miles on Pleasant Valley Road and make a left onto Leisure Lane.

On leaving the winery, continue on Pleasant Valley Road in the direction of Sacramento until it ends at Mother Lode Drive. Turn left onto Mother Lode and follow it into Shingle Springs, where you can access Highway 50 again.

Hike 42 (B) - Jenkinson Lake South Shore Trail
Sly Park, CA

Difficulty: 1

Distance: 8.5-mile loop around the lake, or just do a portion
(i.e., 3.0 miles to bridge at east end of the lake)

Elevation: Flat trail around lake, about 100 feet
change in elevation overall

Directions: Heading East on Highway 50, take the second Pollock Pines exit (Exit 60) for Sly Park Road. At the end of the off-ramp, turn right onto Sly Park Road and travel 4.6 miles to Mormon Emigrant Trail., and make a left. Go 0.8 mile to the trailhead and to a small parking area on your right. If the parking is full, return towards Sly Park Road where more areas are available.

Description: Compared to the Shoreline Trail (Hike 42 A), this is the more wooded and secluded part of the loop trail around Jenkinson Lake. From the trailhead, you head in a counter-clockwise direction along the lake's shore. Currently there work is being done at the trailhead area, fencing around the spillway and redirecting the start of the trail from a service road. Signage is currently temporary, but the trailhead should be well marked by summer, 2008.

Follow signs for hikers, ignoring spurs higher above the lake level for horses. After about 3.0 miles, you will reach a bridge crossing the inlet stream and make it to the sunny side of the lake. There are plenty of places here for a nice lunch break. With shorter days, and colder mornings, at this time of the year it would be difficult to do the entire loop in a single day, so choose between the Shoreline Trail and the South Shore Trail for a nice day hike.

Share with: Bikers

Hike 43 - Codfish Creek Falls Trail
Weimar, CA

Difficulty: 1
Distance: 3.4 miles roundtrip
Elevations: Relatively flat trail with 150' elevation gain
Features: 40-foot waterfall, good family hike

Directions: Take I-80 10 miles east of Auburn, to the second Weimar exit – Weimar Cross Road. Turn right onto Ponderosa Way for 5.7 miles and you will come to the Ponderosa Bridge crossing the North Fork American River. Do not cross this bridge, but turn around and park along the river's side of the road. The trail starts beyond the parking area, going downstream on the north side of the river (again do not cross the bridge to reach the trailhead).

> **Warnings:** *The last 2.4 miles of Ponderosa Way is a graded dirt road descending to the river bottom, and depending on the weather, it can be a rough, slow drive. A 4-wheel drive or high-clearance vehicle is recommended.*

Description: Codfish Creek Falls is a trail everyone can easily enjoy, including small children. It is also an interpretive trail with 14 trail markers pointing out native plants, trees, and wildflowers, and spots for possibly seeing or hearing birds along the river.

The first mile follows along the river before bending away to the right to reach Codfish Creek in another 0.7 mile. At the creek, you will find the falls, wonderful rocks and pools of water, and Marker #14. This is a great picnic and photography spot. There is also a spur trail available to take you to the top of the falls (worth the effort). You will find this spur a short distance back on the main trail as it takes off up the hill.

On your return hike, take time to follow one of the side trails down to the river to enjoy the scenery. Across the river, you can see remnants from the dredge mining of long ago.

Notes: A brochure detailing what you can see at each of the trail markers is not always available at the trailhead. You may want to stop first in Auburn (501 El Dorado St.) to pick one up (or call at 530-885-4527). If their office is closed, you may find a brochure at the California Welcome Center 13411 Lincoln Way (also in Auburn 530-887-2111).

If you do not obtain a brochure, the following identifies the trail markers on the hike.

(1) Manzanita

(2) Canyon Live Oak

(3) A Dipper or Merganser

(4) A California Bay shrub, Dutchman's
      Pipevine, and a Manroot vine

(5) Buck Brush, Buckeye, and Toyon

(6) Interior Live Oak and Goldback Fern

(7) Redbud

(8) Black Oak

(9) Ponderosa Pine

(10) Grey (or digger) Pine

(11) Various wildflowers in the spring, including Lupine,
      California Poppy, Lace Pod, and Larkspur

(12) Douglas fir and the Pacific Madrone
      with its reddish brown bark

(13) The call of the Hutton's Vireo bird

(14) The White Alder and other plants at the creek suited for
      a riparian (water) environment with year round water.

Hike 44 – El Dorado Trail (A)
Placerville, CA

Difficulty: 2
Distance: 5.5 miles round trip
Elevation: 380 feet ascent from trailhead to end of trail

Warning: Parking is limited at the trailhead.

Directions: From Placerville, drive east on Highway 50 about 4.0 miles to the Still Meadows Road exit, into the Apple Café parking lot (no dogs allowed in their outdoor patio). Immediately turn left in the parking lot onto Still Meadows Road and follow it down the hill 0.3 mile to the trail.

Description: The next time you want a light cardio workout, instead of heading to the gym, try out this hike and enjoy the outdoors. The El Dorado Trail runs 6.5 miles. It has both paved (3.1 miles) and unpaved sections (3.4 miles) and is multi-use, serving hikers, bikers, and equestrians.

At the trailhead, choose the route heading uphill towards Camino (the other direction takes you back down towards Placerville.) This is a pleasant 2.75-mile journey with a steady rise the entire way. You will enjoy some great views to the south once you get past the first 1.5 miles bordered by private property (and barking dogs).

There are three benches along the route and numerous seasonal streams. The last mile is definitely the prettiest for viewing, and with the solitude, you can pick up more of the sounds of nature. Along one of the streams in a meadow of willows, I enjoyed the song of the red-winged blackbirds perched throughout the area. Just before the end of the trail, there is a bench making for a perfect lunch spot before you turn around to head back to your car.

For less ambitious choices, head downhill back towards Placerville at the trailhead instead. On this more peaceful route, with a 300-foot elevation change, you will pick up the paved trail in about 1.0 mile. Continuing in that direction, you will come to an overpass crossing Highway 50. In about 2 miles, you will reach the county trailhead for El Dorado Trail (with portable toilets). You could picnic here and turn around.

After the hike, continue up Highway 50 East a short distance to Apple Hill. Take the Carson Road exit (this is a left turn from the highway). There are many farms to visit in Apple Hill, as well as wineries and fruit stands to enjoy. Try a visit to Kids, Inc. for a "walk around" pie (left on Carson Road, then right onto North Canyon Road). They also have a short nature trail there in case your day hike was just not enough. Grandpa's Cellar on Cable Road also has a nature trail. For a winery, try Madrona Vineyards on High Hill Road. Stop in and say "Hi" to owner, Paul, a fellow hiking enthusiast.

Note: For a brochure and trail map for **El Dorado Trail**, visit their website at www.eldoradotrail.org and download the information before your hike.

Share with: Bikers

Hike 44 – El Dorado Trail (B)
Placerville, CA

Difficulty: 1

Distance: 4.0 miles round trip

Directions: Instead of parking at the Still Meadows Road trailhead, drive to the county trailhead (Highway 50 to the Smith Flat Road exit in Placerville to Jacquier Road).

Description: You head from the park 0.1 mile down Jacquier Road to the paved El Dorado Trail running 2.0 miles to the Placerville Station. The paved portion is an easy walk and dotted with benches, flowers, and memorials for those who have donated their efforts to this trail in memory of friends and relatives. It is nicely shaded and includes some pretty views.

Another option is to start from the county trailhead and head east, uphill. This is a pleasant paved stretch of the trail, with a freeway pedestrian crossing. Shortly after crossing the freeway, the pavement will end but the trail continues 3.4 miles to the other end.

DECEMBER

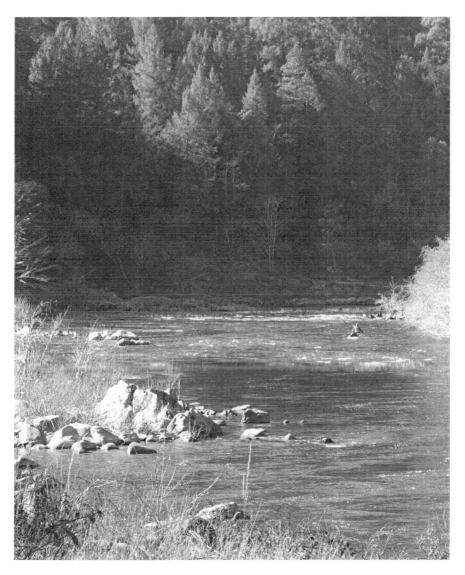

South Fork American River from Red Shack Trail

DECEMBER

With the end of the year, the hikes are closer to home, but with a nice variety of difficulty levels from '2' to '4'. The most difficult is the Red Shack Trail hike down to the American River and then the strenuous 850-foot climb back up. You return to Olmstead Loop, but do the portion you shortcut in May, pass by an interesting stand of boulders known as Pointed Rocks, and journey down to "No Hands Bridge."

Then you will return to Falcon Crest in El Dorado Hills, but hike an entirely different portion of the trail, ending at New York Creek. End the month with a drive towards Foresthill and hike the Foresthill Divide Loop. For those with physical limitations, there are less ambitious options on the New York Creek, Red Shack, and Pointed Rocks trail descriptions.

Hike 45 - New York Creek
El Dorado Hills, CA

Difficulty: 2

Distance: 3.5 miles to New York Creek

Elevation: Mostly rolling hike with a total of 200 feet elevation change, including a couple 50-foot ascents

Warning: *Poison Oak (although it has dropped its leaves, the stick-like branches can still give you poison oak). Do not attempt this hike in the spring or summer when the poison oak covers the trail.*

Directions: To reach the parking area, from Green Valley Road turn south onto Salmon Falls Road and travel 2.9 miles to find the gravel parking area on your left, signed as Falcon Crest. (From Highway 50 you can take the El Dorado Hills Boulevard exit and go north 4.2 miles to Green Valley Road. Cross Green Valley Road at the signal, and then it becomes Salmon Falls Road).

Description: Enjoy a stroll in the foothills and take in some great views along the South Fork American River portion of Folsom Lake. This hike takes you to New York Creek and lets you see where it flows into the river. Enjoy the creek's riparian habitat when you stop for your lunch break. This is a great time of the year for this journey. The hills are beginning to turn green; the poison oak has lost its leaves; the water is low for you to see the inflows more easily; and, the weather is cool for a perfect hiking experience. It is both peaceful and active, with quail and jackrabbits scurrying around, no doubt making last-minute preparations for winter.

From the parking area, find the trailhead marker on your left beside the green service gate. This is the marker for the Monte Vista Trail

North. In a short distance (about 250 feet), you will reach a junction and a sign for Monte Vista Trail South to the left and Monte Vista Trail North straight ahead. Continue straight here and follow the trail up to a ridge and open area. At the open area (field of thistle and other weeds), the trail goes left.

In a short distance, locate the picnic area on your left at the apex of the ridge. This is a good resting spot with potable water and some photographic views of the surrounding hills and homes. From the picnic area, continue down the trail to another junction signed Monte Vista Trail North. Bear left at this junction to go towards New York Creek (not signed).

Continue 0.1 mile to another junction marked only with two green State Park posts. Turn right here and go another 0.1 mile to reach Brown's Ravine Trail. At the intersection with the Brown's Ravine Trail, you want to head left towards the Brown's Ravine Assembly Area (a right turn takes you towards the Old Salmon Fall Assembly Area). From this point, it is approximately 2.9 miles to New York Creek. You will begin to get mile markers for the Brown's Ravine Trail. The first will be at the 14.5-mile mark.

Along the trail, you cross several streams (some dry). You will get your first glimpse of the lake, and perhaps a lone heron at water's edge resting on a protruding stump. At the 13-mile marker, you will see New York Creek on your right. Follow the trail now for less than a mile and you will come to where it crosses the creek. This is your turnaround (unless you wish to go further). You will find this a great picnic and photography spot.

Return on Brown's Ravine Trail until you reach the "Monte Vista Trail South (.6)" Sign. Turn right here and continue until you reach two State Park markers. The one on the left points left to Potable Water. The one on the right is signed Monte Vista South and points right to Potable Water. Turn right here and continue on the dirt road.

At the final intersection (not signed), again turn right and follow the service road up to the green gate and the parking area.

Less Ambitious Option: Stop at the picnic area and then turn around to return to your car.

Share with: Horses

Hike 46 - Pointed Rocks Trail to No Hands Bridge
Olmstead Loop
Auburn State Recreation Area

Difficulty: 3

Distance: 6.5-mile loop

Elevation: 1000 feet elevation change, but generally a rolling hike except for steep 800-foot descent and then the return ascent

Warning: 0.9- mile steep descent

Directions: On Highway 49 in Cool, turn on Saint Florian Court at the fire station and find the parking area just behind it. The first level of parking is for cars, and the upper parking area is for horse trailers. If you are coming from Auburn, it is a right turn just before the fire station and the Stop sign. Coming from Coloma, make a left turn just after the Stop sign in Cool and the fire station.

Description: I believe this is the most scenic route via "No Hands Bridge." If you were to do this hike in the reverse direction, it would rate a '5' in difficulty. You will be treated with some great vistas and perfect trail conditions in December.

You start by parking behind the firehouse in Cool off Highway 49. Park in the first gravel lot behind the station (the second lot is for horse trailers). This is the trailhead for the Olmstead Loop Trail.

Start the loop in reverse direction, so cross the street to enter the trail at its actual end (the 9.0-mile mark). Follow the trail beside Highway 49 for a short while before it heads west away from the road and into the rolling foothills. You will pass four trail junctions on your way to Pointed Rocks. Follow the green State Park post marker at each junction to stay on the Olmstead Loop Trail.

After 1.3 miles, you will see a field of boulders known as Pointed Rocks. Here you can rest and enjoy the Sierra views and the colorful lichen covering on the rocks. As you continue beyond here, the distant views are even more photogenic. Then in a short while, you will come to the junction with Training Hill Trail.

You will leave Olmstead Loop here and take this trail to the right. You will reach a sign warning of a 0.9-mile steep downhill. On the way down, enjoy the coolness of pine cover and great views of Foresthill Bridge, the distant mountains, and the hillside homes in Auburn. Take the descent slowly and enjoy.

At trail's end, you will come to "No Hands Bridge" (local name for Mountain Quarries Railroad Bridge credited to equestrians crossing it with hands off the reins) crossing the North Fork American River and a pleasant resting spot. Just before the bridge, there is a steep spur trail down to the river and a very nice beach for a picnic and a rest. After your lunch, take time to walk across the bridge. There is a marker at the far end giving you historical information about the bridge.

When ready for the return trip, start on the same route from "No Hands Bridge" back up the hill. In a short distance, you will come to a junction. The sign shows Training Hill Trail straight and the Western States Trail (WST) left, with Cool 3.3 miles away. Take the left turn here and continue following signs in the direction towards Cool. The WST trail joins the Wendell T. Robie Trail. Stay on this trail and in the direction of Cool (pass by the junction for Short Cut Trail). For a while, the trail follows the canyon side bordering the highway, and it is noisy and very cool. Then it turns away, and you will reach a more open terrain dotted by deciduous oaks with their leaves turning colors.

At the 7.5-mile state marker, veer left along an old fence line and follow this trail for a short while until you emerge back onto Olmstead Loop. Go left here and retrace your route back to the parking area.

After the Hike: For some authentic Mexican food, try the Main Street Café & Grill on Highway 49 in Cool (530) 888-6209.

Less Ambitious Option: Just hike to Pointed Rocks and then turn around there. Do not attempt the Training Hill Descent unless you are sure of your balance. Once you return to your car, drive along Highway 49 towards Auburn to the parking area for "No Hands Bridge". This area is opposite the river's side of Highway 49, just before crossing over the river. Walk in to the bridge from here.

Share with: Horses

Hike 47 - Red Shack Trail
Placerville

Difficulty: 4

Distance: 3.0 miles roundtrip

Elevation: Downhill going to the river, but
steep return ascent of 850 feet

Directions: On Highway 49 between Coloma and Placerville, find the Red Shack produce stand and the parking area for the trail across the highway. From Coloma, you go 5.6 miles on Highway 40 towards Placerville to reach the trail. Coming into Placerville from Sacramento on Highway 50, turn left at Spring Street (second light) and go 3.5 miles on Highway 49 towards Coloma.

Description: This is a 1.5 mile hike down to the South Fork American River with an elevation drop of about 850 feet, so be prepared to make an 850-foot ascent over 1.5 miles on the return trip. There are enough switchbacks on the old dirt road used for a trail to ease the climb somewhat. Still, I would rate this hike a '4' in difficulty – it is not for those with a weak heart.

It takes about 30 minutes down the canyon to the river and 35 minutes back up to the trailhead. Just before reaching the bottom of the trail, you cross an old ditch once used for conducting water from Chili Bar to Lotus (Coloma-Lotus Ranch Ditch). Plan on spending time at the river to take pictures, watch kayakers, and enjoy a picnic lunch in the sun before your return trip.

After the hike, you can read the historical marker a few feet away from the parking area, to learn about the Luse Ditch Flume, and then continue on Highway 49 into Placerville and a walk on Main Street. (Cross Highway 50 at the light in Placerville, then turn left and continue straight to Main Street while Highway 49 will wind away to the right.)

December is a great month on Main Street for finding unique Christmas gifts, tasting some cheese from Dedrick's along with wine or beer from The Wine Smith. At Placerville News, you can find topographical maps and books on California wildflowers. During December weekends, the city of Placerville offers free stagecoach rides, live music, and costumed actors representing the "Old Hangtown" times of the 1850's.

Less Ambitious Option: Visit the Red Shack trailhead and read the historical marker, then make your way to Main Street in Placerville for a pleasant stroll and shopping.

Hike 48 - Foresthill Divide Loop Trail
Foresthill, CA

Difficulty: 2

Distance: 8.2-mile loop

Elevation: Undulating hike with mostly 50-100 foot ascents, and two 200-foot ascents

Directions: From the Foresthill Bridge, continue east on Foresthill Road 7.0 miles to the large parking area on the left (this is 0.2 mile past the right turn for Driver's Flat Road).

Description: This is a pleasant, cool, loop through wooded foothill terrain, but with enough ascents to make for a rewarding workout. It is also one of the most popular mountain bike rides in Placer County, so be prepared to make way for bikers and horses on busy weekends.

Starting from the parking area, walk through the green gate and just past the portable toilet, you will see the Foresthill Divide Loop Trail starting to the left. The trail starts in a shaded woodland ecosystem with oaks, manzanita, buckeyes, pines, and native brush. At 2.5 miles, the trail crosses the dirt road to Upper Lake Clementine.

Soon you will be walking through a grove of madrones. Continue another 1.3 miles to the end of the first half of the loop (near the end there is a fork to the right – remain on the left, more traveled fork). Here you need to carefully cross Foresthill Road and walk east up the road about 0.5-mile. You will come to another green gate (#119) where you can reenter the trail. After a short distance, you will turn left to continue the loop.

On this 4.0-mile section of the loop, there are open meadows, larger oaks, and more expansive views. After a difficult 200-foot ascent, there is a nice plateau suitable for a lunch spot. From here, you will make a little descent. Along the way, be sure you watch for trail markers, leading you first to the left and then to the right. You will descend to a creek habitat, with grapes, old pear and fig trees, and a nice wood bridge over the seasonal spring. This is the only potential water for your dog on the loop, so be sure to bring water and a way to let your dog get a drink.

A little after leaving the creek, there will be a signed left turn for the trail away from a dirt road. Continue along the loop where it will come out to a road. Turn right onto the road for a minute and then you will see the trail again to your right. The trail will take you to a large parking area above a park entrance and onto Drivers Flat Road. From here, you can walk up the road to Foresthill Road and a short 0.2-mile jaunt back to the parking area, or find the trail again beyond the garbage cans to take you out to Foresthill Road Either way, you need to cross the road carefully to return to your car.

Share with: Bikers

Resources

Before engaging in any hike, gather all available information regarding conditions and availability. Always have the appropriate map and trail information before undertaking any adventure.

Amador Ranger Station – El Dorado National Forest (209) 295-4251 26820 Silver Drive Pioneer, CA 95666 for information on hiking conditions along Highway 88 ((Kirkwood and Carson Pass) and the Mokelumne Wilderness www.fs.fed.us/r5/eldorado/recreation/wild/moke/cpma

Auburn State Recreation Area (530) 885-4527 501 El Dorado Street Auburn, CA 95603 www.parks.ca.gov for hikes along Highway 49 and Foresthill

California Welcome Center (530) 887-2111 13422 Lincoln Way Auburn, CA 95603 for maps and trail suggestions for Auburn State Recreation Area www.visitplacer.com

Crystal Basin (530) 647-5415 for Loon Lake, Bassi Falls, and Gerle Creek hikes

Echo Lakes (530) 659-7207 for water taxi information

El Dorado Trail www.eldoradotrail.org

El Dorado National Forest www.fs.fed.us/r5/eldorado (530) 644-6048

Folsom Lake State Recreation Area (916) 988-0205   7806 Folsom-Auburn Road for a map and information about Folsom Lake trails www.parks.ca.gov

Foresthill Ranger District (530) 367-2224   22830 Foresthill Road www.fs.fed.us/r5/tahoe for brochure to Placer Big Trees

Georgetown Ranger Station (530) 333-4312 for University Falls

Kirkwood Cross Country & Snowshoe Center (209) 258-7248 www.kirkwood.com

Lake Tahoe Basin Management Unit (530) 543-2694   35 College Drive South Lake Tahoe, CA www.fs.fed.us/r5/ltbmu

Lake Tahoe Visitor Center 3.2 miles on Highway 89 after the 89/50 split for day permits into Desolation Wilderness

Marshall Museum & Visitor Center (530) 622-3470 and www.marshallgold.org

Pacific Ranger District (530) 647-5415 Mill Run Road in Fresh Pond off Highway 50 for day-use permits into Desolation Wilderness

Placerville Downtown Association (530) 672-3436 for details of activities on Main Street in December www.cityofplacerville.org

Sly Park Recreation Area for Jenkinson Lake (530) 644-2545 www.eid.org

South Yuba River State Park (530) 432-2546

Tallac Historic Site (530) 541-5227

Taylor Creek Visitor Center (530) 543-2674

Valhalla Arts & Music (530) 541-4975   for upcoming events at Valhalla and the Tallac Historic Site www.valhallatahoe.com

For topographical maps, go to Placerville News at 409 Main Street in Placerville. For a complete map of topography and trails in Desolation Wilderness, visit any REI store. Visit the California Welcome Center in Auburn for a map of the Auburn State Recreation Area.

For day-use permits in Desolation Wilderness, stop on Highway 50 in Fresh Pond at the Mill Run exit for the Pacific Ranger District. During the prime hiking season, permits are generally available at all trailheads, but after the season, you will need to pick one up at the station. For the Mt. Tallac hike in October, there may still be permits at the trailhead, but you can also pick one up at the Lake Tahoe Visitor Center on Highway 89. Permits are required year round.

TRAIL INDEX

Below is general information about the places you hike to in this book. Note that in the book, you hike to Caples Creek in June, but Fall Colors is marked, indicating a place to return to in the fall. Similarly, you hike to University Falls in March to view the falls, but "Swimming" is marked for a possible return trip idea in late summer. All trails will display some wildflowers, but the ones marked have the best displays.

The trails marked for fishing are those I have personally fished with my husband or watched others fish successfully. A number of hikes along the river offer fishing and gold panning opportunities.

Trails marked for physical accessibility are all good hikes for anyone new to exercise, recovering from surgery (with doctor's approval), overweight, or physically handicapped. If you can walk with a cane or a walker, then all of these should be doable for you. If you require a wheelchair, then read the trail description to verify wheelchair accessibility.

Hike	Wildflowers	Fall Colors	Waterfalls	Kid Friendly	Physical Accessibility	Big Trees	Historical Interest	Fishing	Swimming	Views	Gold Panning	Fee
1. Marshall State Park				*	*		*			*	*	*
2. Kirkwood				*								*
3. Pt. Defiance				*			*				*	
4. Cronan Ranch												
5. Sweetwater Creek				*			*			*		
6. Purdon Crossing							*			*	*	
7. Meeks Creek				*								
8. Old Salmon Falls				*								
9. Loon Lake Chalet				*								
10. Peninsula Campground					*							*
11. University Falls			*						*			
12. Bear Falls			*	*								

142

Hike	Wildflowers	Fall Colors	Waterfalls	Kid Friendly	Physical Accessibility	Big Trees	Historical Interest	Fishing	Swimming	Views	Gold Panning	Fee
13. Buttermilk Bend	*			*								
14. Quarry Road				*	*						*	
15. Darrington Bike Trail	*			*								
16. Lake Clementine			*					*	*	*	*	
17. Placer Big Trees				*		*						
18. Olmstead Loop	*											
19. Dave Moore Nature Area	*	*		*	*						*	
20. Independence Trail	*		*	*	*		*			*		
21. Georgetown Nature Area	*			*	*		*					
22. Tallac/Valhalla	*			*	*	*	*			*		
23. Caples Creek		*	*			*			*	*		
24. Horsetail Falls			*							*		*

143

Hike	Wildflowers	Fall Colors	Waterfalls	Kid Friendly	Physical Accessibility	Big Trees	Historical Interest	Fishing	Swimming	Views	Gold Panning	Fee
25. Bassi Falls			*	*								
26. Umpa Lake			*					*	*			
27. Maud Lake	*	*						*				
28. Winnemucca/ Round Top	*							*		*		*
29. Boomerang Lake								*	*			
30. Lake Sylvia	*	*	*					*	*	*		
31. Dardanelles Lake								*				
32. Shealor Lake								*	*	*		
33. Lover's Leap										*		
34. Pearl Lake										*		
35. Gertrude Lake								*				
36. Gerle Creek				*	*		*					

144

Hike	Wildflowers	Fall Colors	Waterfalls	Kid Friendly	Physical Accessibility	Big Trees	Historical Interest	Fishing	Swimming	Views	Gold Panning	Fee
37. Tamarack/Ralston/Cagwin								*	*	*		
38. Lake Margaret		*						*		*		
39. Nevada Beach				*	*							
40. Mt. Tallac via Floating Is.		*								*		
41. Grouse/Hemlock/Smith								*		*		
42. Jenkinson Lake				*	*			*	*			
43. Codfish Creek Falls		*	*	*								
44. El Dorado Trail												
45. New York Creek				*						*		
46. Pointed Rocks										*		
47. Red Shack							*				*	
48. Foresthill Divide Loop										*		

Bikes Trails

Camp Richardson – bike trail along Lake Tahoe Hike 22

Cronan Ranch – mountain bike trail to the South Fork American River   Hike 4

Darrington Trail from Salmon Falls Bridge – mountain bike trail to Peninsula Campground   Hike 15   (reverse direction from Hike 10)

El Dorado Trail – paved and unpaved portions in Placerville   Hike 44

Foresthill Divide Loop – popular mountain bike trail in Placer County Hike 48

Jenkinson Lake – trail around lake in Sly Park   Hike 42 (the South Shore portion requires a mountain bike)

Lake Clementine – trail from the American River confluence along the North Fork to the dam at Lake Clementine   Hike 16

Olmstead Loop – loop trail for mountain bikes with creek crossings and lots of hills and views   Hike 18

Purdon Crossing – mountain bike trail along the South Fork Yuba River   Hike 6

Quarry Road – mountain bike trail along the Middle Fork American River   Hike 14

Sweetwater Creek – mountain bike trail along the South Fork American River portion of Folsom Lake   Hike 5

No bikes are allowed in Desolation Wilderness

EQUESTRIAN TRAILS

Horses and pack animals are allowed on most trails within Desolation Wilderness. Always yield to these animals.

Caples Creek trail – mostly populated by hikers, but you will see an occasional horse or motorized two-wheelers on parts of the trail   Hike 23

Cronan Ranch – this is a very popular equestrian site with miles of horse trails (horses outnumber hikers)   Hike 4

Olmstead Loop trail and the trail to **No Hands Bridge** both are popular with equestrians Hikes 18 and 46

New York Creek – you can go 12 miles beyond the described hike's destination to New York Creek and continue to Brown's Ravine at Folsom Lake and on to the Dam   Hike 45

Peninsula Campground – this is the better starting end of the Darrington Trail for horses (rather than the Salmon Falls Bridge starting point)   Hike 10

South Yuba Trail/Purdon Crossing – primarily a hiking or biking trail, you can also see horses here   Hike 6

GLOSSARY

bar: a raised area in a river formed by sand and boulders backing up the water above it and forming a pool

blazes: man-made cuts in trees above eye-level to mark a trail

Desolation Wilderness: an area of approximately 100 square miles in the Sierra Nevada generally accessible for hiking from July to November; day use permits are required to enter the wilderness

ducks: conspicuous piles of about three to five rocks to mark a trail

elevation: in this book the elevation refers to the feet gained from the lowest point to the highest point of the trail; this is not a calculation of total vertical feet climbed – which is generally greater due to the undulating terrain of most hikes

Foresthill Bridge: designed to span the proposed reservoir created with the Auburn Dam, the 2,248-foot long bridge stands 730 feet high; work stopped on the dam project in 1976 leaving the bridge as an enduring reminder and the tallest bridge in California

fork: a split in the trail with two equal-looking trails taking off (not a spur), one to the right and the other to the left usually without markings; refer to a good map or trail description to take the correct fork

loop trail: a loop trail allows you to return from the trail's destination on a different route from which you came; whenever you can, return to a loop hike and do in the reverse direction to pick up different sites

riparian: an environment for vegetation adapted to year-round water as you would find along a creek or river

service gate: an iron gate crossing the road leading from a trailhead; always leave access to the gate available for emergency or service vehicles

spur trail: a minor footpath taking off from the main trail to lead you to a specific site such as the river or a viewing spot before you return to the main trail

topographic map: area map showing elevation contour lines representing every 40-foot elevation change (every 200-foot line being darker) creating an easy way to judge the grade steepness by the line density

trailhead: the starting point for the hike, usually adjacent to the parking area

ups and downs: undulating foothill terrain with trail dropping down 10-100 feet and then climbing back up 10-100 feet for no elevation change but vertical feet climbed

Western States Trail: a 100-mile endurance run from Squaw Valley in Lake Tahoe to Auburn

REFERENCES

Blackwell, Laird R. *Wildflowers of the Sierra Nevada and the Central Valley.* Edmonton, AB: Lone Pine Publishing, 1999.

Peterson, Tom. *Georgetown Hiking Trails.* Georgetown, CA: Tom Peterson, 2005.

Schaffer, Jeffrey P. *Desolation Wilderness and the South Lake Tahoe Basin.* Berkeley, CA: Wilderness Press, 2003.

Soares, Marc J. *Snowshoe Routes: Northern California.* Seattle, WA: The Mountaineers Books, 2002.

Soares, Marc J. *75 Year-Round Hikes in Northern California.* Seattle, WA: The Mountaineers Books, 2000.

Index

About the Author

Looking for a way to exercise her dog, Toots, Debbi Preston started hiking in Desolation Wilderness in 2003. They both enjoyed the experience, but when the snow came to the mountains, their hiking trips ended. As soon as the trails cleared in 2004, they were back to the mountains, exploring hikes to various alpine lakes.

This time, when the snow returned, hiking was too much of a passion to stop and wait five or six months to return to the mountains. Debbi started looking in books for winter and spring trail possibilities, but most were too far away for a day trip or did not allow dogs. She expanded her search for foothill trails by talking with friends, finding web sites on hiking, studying maps, visiting ranger stations and park headquarters, and looking for trailheads while driving.

Over the next three years, Debbi found suitable trails for each month of the year. She wanted trails that rewarded the hiker with great views, wildflowers, waterfalls, or historic interest. She also liked places without any fees. To extend the hiking season in the mountains, she added snowshoeing in the winter. Then, wanting her mother to join in some outings, she looked for places with access for those with physical limitations. She scaled down some hikes to match her mother's capabilities, and found others that would accommodate a walker.

Debbi added photography to her outings, and turned some of the scenes into oil paintings. One summer she concentrated on studying wildflowers by photographing and then identifying and organizing them by color and number of petals. A credentialed community college teacher, Debbi was also passionate about sharing her knowledge with others and teaching the rewards of hiking. With the encouragement of her husband, Jeff, she organized the hikes into this book.

CPSIA information can be obtained at www.ICGtesting.com
Printed in the USA
LVOW101741010412

275521LV00002B/2/P